NUTRITION ILLUSION

Why Plant-Based Diets Are Not What They Seem To Be

Emmanuel Lafrance

ect or indirect, that are incurred as a result of the use of the information contained within this document, including, but not limited to, errors, omissions, or inaccuracies.

TABLE OF CONTENTS

INTRODUCTION

Plants are not what they seem to be. Common household plants, such as desk cacti and decorative flowers, are not the issue I'm about to discuss with you. The plants we eat—everything from the potato you enjoy cut up into fries or mashed and served with gravy, to the leafy greens you add to your protein shakes—are not all that we have been told to believe. The popularity of plant-based diets has led to an increase in the demand for plant foods, plant-based meat substitutes, and plant-based milks. While enjoying plant foods as part of a balanced, well-maintained diet is not necessarily harmful, their prevalence does raise some concerns. The way we view plant-based diets and their long-reaching effect on the environment, in general, has been simplified to such an extent that some significant issues are being overlooked.

First, we have forgotten where the plant foods we enjoy today have come from. Generations of selective breeding and genetic engineering have created an abundance of plant foods, which our early ancestors would not be able to recognize. In fact, they might even be less nutritionally viable than the plant foods our early ancestors previously enjoyed. The plants we eat are simply not what they used to be. Watermelons have been bred to be bigger, fuller, and juicier. While they might make a cooing summer snack and a low-calorie option for those trying to lose weight, they do not contain the levels of nutrients you might expect. The same is true of all plant foods. While spinach is advertised as a "source of iron" and beans are an "alternative source of protein," there are hidden factors we ignore. In recent years, food scientists have been studying a phenomenon known as antinutrients. Later in this book I will go into more detail about what these are.

Second, the modern food supply is grown in such a way that is very detrimental to the environment. The steady expanse of farming for food causes innumerable environmental problems. Monocultural farming, for example, is a practice which leads to increased risk of pests, degradation of soil, and weak crop yields. This has led to an increased reliance on synthetic chemical pesticides and fertilizers, residue of which can be found on the plant foods you might buy at the grocery store. And it doesn't stop there. The level of tillage required to break up the soil for the sowing season damages the structure of the soil, preventing plants from growing strong, deep roots and absorbing moisture from the ground. This is just a fraction of the problems caused by tilling. And this is not to speak of the problems caused to local water supplies from the runoff of fertilizers and groundwater. But we'll get to that.

Third, and this is not addressed enough, plant foods are an inadequate source of nutrition. Spinach does not contain nearly enough iron to sustain a person or assist with the body's processes, nor do carrots help with the health of your eyes. While genetic engineering has been helpful in producing crops with large yields, it has come at the cost of the plant's nutritional value. Plants need a lot of energy and nutrition in order to thrive and their needs are not being met with modern farming standards. As a result, the plants we are given to eat do not contain the essential vitamins and minerals to meet the demands of the human body. Protein, for example, is a difficult source to come by for most people who eat a plant-based diet. Legumes, nuts, mushrooms, and beans are all advertised as great alternatives to lean red meat, poultry, and fish but none of these contain the omega-3 fatty acids the body needs for cellular or joint health. Plants do contain a hefty amount of fiber, which is great for maintaining bowel health but this does nothing if the body cannot absorb what little nutrients that have been received from plants.

Fourth, as I mentioned before, the rise in interest regarding antinutrients has yielded some interesting information. Phytic acid, protease inhibitors, and lectins all play vital roles in the life cycle of plants, particularly in the seedling and early growing stages but, as the plants are being harvested, trace amounts remain. These trace amounts inevitably become more prevalent in larger portions. A single bean, for example, contains a small amount of phytic acid, which will not do that much in the way of preventing your body from gaining nutrition. However, in a larger serving of, say, 100g, that phytic acid is suddenly compounded and its effects become more noticeable. We will go into detail about the different types of antinutrients later on. For now, know that they prevent the absorption of certain essential nutrients, especially minerals and it can also damage your gut lining. There are ways to reduce the levels of antinutrients present in your plant foods but, again, that is a topic for a later chapter.

Fifth, while it is entirely possible to build muscle on a plant-based diet, it is extremely difficult. Plant-based meat substitutes, such as soy steaks and pea protein burgers, contain more carbohydrates, fat, and salt than a cut of beef or chicken breast. The body needs protein for a variety of processes. Not only does it help with injury repair, protein also assists with muscular hypertrophy. This is colloquially known as "gains." Bodybuilders, wrestlers, and anyone who relies on strong muscles understands the importance of protein in their diet. Protein shakes exist as a supplement, not as a meal replacement. However, the fitness and diet industry has taken the opportunity to tout protein shakes which offer "everything you need." I will go into detail later as to why this is not the case. Protein shakes help to increase your intake of protein but they are not to be relied upon. Some brands might claim that their shakes are blended with all the amino acids your body needs. This is not the case. At best, these types of protein shakes are expensive smoothie mixes. More legitimate brands which design their protein shakes according to the needs of health and fitness enthusiasts are healthier and along the right track of what the body needs. Generally speaking, there are two sources of protein: animal-based and plant-based. All animal protein, contained in fish and eggs for example, is considered a complete protein because it has all 9 essential amino acids in elevated numbers. Some plant-based proteins, however, are incomplete protein which means they are lacking in at least 1 essential amino acid. Moreover, not all plant proteins are digested and used by the human body, but we will get to the "why" later on.

Sixth, anyone who consumes a diet heavy on plant products will experience a variety of symptoms. The intensity of these symptoms entirely depends on how much plant foods who consume. People who eat "plant-based" or vegans will experience these symptoms at the fullest degree. For the sake of this book, let's get in the shoes of a standard American dieter starting a vegan diet. At first, the change in diet, the increase in Vitamin C and sudden influx of fiber and "lighter" foods will leave the person feeling a little healthier. As the body processes everything it is being given, it will start to release more energy and you will feel more awake and alert. Unfortunately, this will cease after just a few weeks. For both men and women, muscle loss is not uncommon in the months following the change to a plant-based diet. Men might experience increased hair loss while women will start to develop hormonal inconsistencies. These are just the lesser symptoms. Tooth decay, gut problems, accelerated fat gain and muscle loss will also be explored in due time. Any change in diet is likely to have its negative side effects. The first two weeks of the keto diet are known as "keto flu" because the body is adjusting to ketosis and you are likely to experience flu-like symptoms (headache, nausea, slight fever, etc.) during those two weeks. I'd argue that the first few weeks of a plant-based diet are the inverse of keto flu, with the months that follow being an amplified variant. You also stand to lose a lot of nutrition from plant-based diets. In order to prevent this, increased supplementation is required. Iron deficiencies are common in vegans and vegetarians, although the latter of these two have more sources available to them.

Seventh, although I am writing this book to expose and

explore the damages caused by plant foods, I recognize that my diet is not suited to everyone. I follow a keto plan which is heavy on meats and fats with a small amount of plant foods. For this reason, I would like to explore some ways in which you can get the most out of your plants. A huge part of this involves breaking down and degrading the levels of antinutrients you will find. Everyday cooking techniques such as boiling, frying, and even fermentation are excellent ways of denaturing the structures of antinutrients and releasing other nutrients which might be hiding within the plant. Although antinutrients are a very real problem, they can be resolved quite easily. Additionally, growing your own food is a great way to gain control of your diet. This also cuts down on the amount of pesticides required and offers the option to grow varieties you might prefer. If growing your own plant foods is not viable for you, finding a local farm and buying organic is a great way to support your local economy.

Eighth, and lastly, we should be a lot more mindful about our diets. As the food, fitness, and health industries have grown, we have lost our understanding of nutrition and how it relates to our overall health and wellbeing. There are a variety of diets which can be categorized as either animal-based or plant-based. Of the animal-based diets, you have the options of pescetarianism, the Mediterranean diet, the ketogenic diet and carnivore diet, among other options. On the plant-based side of the spectrum, you have the standard vegetarianism and veganism, although flexitarianism and some forms of the keto diet are arguably plant-based. At the end of this book, we will explore a few diet options. The purpose of this chapter will be to help you make an informed decision about your diet. That being said, no two people will ever have the same diet. A standard American diet does not suit everyone, just like a plant-based diet does not suit me. For this reason, I advise seeking the advice of a dietician or nutritionist before embarking on a brand new dietary venture.

I have spent the last 5 years studying nutrition. It's a fascinating subject and I have enjoyed every moment of it. After about a year, I decided to go vegetarian to see what all the fuss was about. Within the first 3 months, I learned a few critical things about my body. Most notably that it is not suited for a plant-based diet. Next, I tried the ketogenic diet. After 6 months, I learned something new: it made me feel good. The increased intake of protein and fat helped my body run more efficiently. After this discovery, I decided to push it a little further and subsisted on a carnivorous diet for 2 years. Today, I still eat a mostly meat-based diet, although I have been known to indulge in plant foods from time to time.

In terms of the things I learned about my body during my short stint as a vegetarian, I noticed that my skin broke out even more. We've all had that one pimple that we just can't shake or that patch of skin that gets so dry that we become obsessed with trying to cure it as quickly as we can. This was me while I was vegetarian. My skin was so bad that I was obsessed with trying to cure it and I knew that it was something to do with my diet. The more I studied nutrition, the more certain I became. After a while, I made the connection between my diet and my skin problems. Therefore, I soon went back on my "drawing board" to create my new diet. Now, if you're reading this, you have probably had similar experiences. Maybe you've tried a carnivorous diet and struggled to maintain it or you've tried a plant-based diet and had such low energy that you could barely move out of bed. I've been on both ends of the dietary spectrum. Not everyone has access to the same level of professional nutritional knowledge that I do. For this reason, my goal is to bring some clarity to the science of nutrition and dieting. I will be using scientific terminology and wherever I do use a word you are unfamiliar with, I will break it down and make it simple. This is something I have been passionate about for a long time and I would be delighted to share my knowledge with you.

A community

If you want to be part of a likeminded community, you can join our facebook group Nutrition Delusion where we share plenty of interresting facts and edifying stories. My books will also be available at a discounted price if you join the facebook group.

Plus, you can directly go to my website:
www.nutritiondelusion.com
to get your very own free copy of my <u>7 lies About Food</u> list. All you have to do is enter your name and email address and you will receive your free copy in your emails. Don't forget to check in your junk mails :)

Also, please don't forget to **leave a review** on Amazon. Every review helps authors like me reach more people.

CHAPTER 1: PLANTS ARE NOT WHAT THEY USED TO BE

Evolution is the scientific theory of heritable change according to an organism's surroundings. It has persisted for millennia, perfectly sculpting humans, animals, and plants within their given genes to thrive in their environments. As humanity progressed, so did our love of food and our ability to grow it for ourselves. Farming itself evolved, enabling us to produce large quantities of food within the growing season and, as food preservation techniques evolved, so have the plants we have come to enjoy on a daily basis. Bioengineering was developed to study and develop hardier crops for future planting, ostensibly to improve the nutritional quality of the crop.

Genetic engineering and selective breeding are both valuable tools in bioengineering. Through this, we have been able to create larger crop yields as well as shorten the growing season. Selective breeding is the process used by humans to create a new organism with desirable characteristics. The "parent" organisms are selected based on specific characteristics. Take, for example, tomatoes. One parent plant might have a rich red color but grows slowly, while the other parent plant grows quickly but does not have the rich red color. Bioengineers splice the DNA of each plant and extract the desirable genes from each, then combine them to create a new type of plant. These plants are therefore known as "genetically modified organisms" or GMOs.

GMOs are not necessarily a bad thing. If anything, we can say that they're one of the best things humans have developed in recent years. Without them, we would not have the abundance of food sources that we have. Some GMOs have been developed to be more nutritious than what you would typically find in the wild, while others have been bred to be more resistant to particular diseases. Humans have been able to achieve a lot over the last few thousand years when it comes to sustainable crop yields and developments in farming. One might even suggest that without GMOs, we might struggle significantly to maintain the quality of life and availability many of us have become accustomed to.

The problem with GMOs is not that they're bad for us. As I've mentioned, some might be better for us than what we might be able to find in the wild. However, most GMO crops are treated with pesticides, which contain harmful chemical byproducts. Another problem with GMOs, which might surprise you, is the fact that they cannot survive in the wild. They can't stand up on their own to certain fungi or pests, so they need to be treated with strong pesticides and fungicides to keep them healthy and alive. They are entirely dependent on humans for their survival and while some

GMO plants are more nutritious, the majority of the GMOs we find for sale at the local grocery store might be less nutrient-dense than we need them to be.

Man-Made Plants

If you were to go back in time 10,000 years ago and survey the flora and fauna, you would find the ancestor plants of many of the varieties we enjoy today. These would mostly be in the form of berries, roots, nuts, and beans. That is not to say, however, that these plants are the same as what you would find in the local grocery store. In fact, these plants would likely be more nutrient-dense and harder to come by. Foraging, in addition to hunting, was a common means by which early hominids were able to gather food. You might think that our ancient ancestors might look at us now, with sustenance in such abundance, and say that we are doing well. However, the purpose of eating food is to provide fuel and essential nutrients for the body. Would our ancient ancestors be surprised to learn that the plants we eat might be less nutritious than the food they gathered and farmed?

Veggies

Here is a list of common vegetables. What is the one thing you think they have in common?

- Brussels Sprouts
- Broccoli
- Kale

- Kohlrabi
- Cauliflower
- Cabbage

If your guess was that they're all delicious, nutritious green veggies that can be made into a variety of meals, you'd be somewhat right. That's just one answer, though. All 6 of these vegetables, while delicious when appropriately prepared, are related to each other by a single parent plant. Brassica oleracea, though you may not have ever heard of it, is definitely in your diet in some form or another. It's most commonly known as the wild mustard plant and the 6 vegetables listed above are its cultivars. A cultivar is simply a subspecies of one plant. Kohlrabi is a cultivar of the wild mustard stem, cauliflower and broccoli were cultivated from the flower buds.

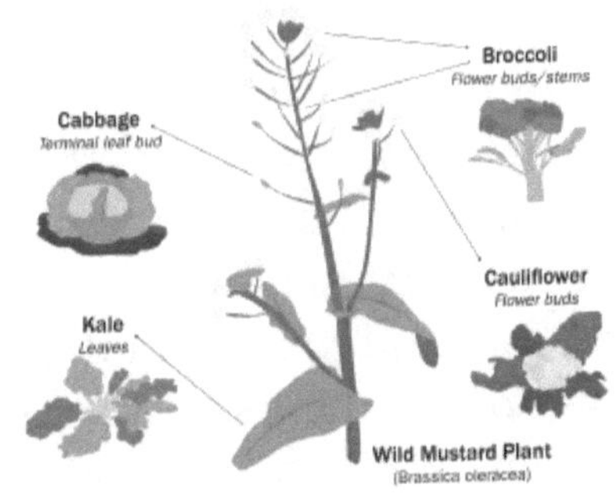

By selecting the right leaf or part of the stem, new subspecies can be created. Returning to the example of broccoli, selecting the largest flower buds and cultivating them was how this bulky green vegetable began its evolution. This can even be seen to this day; when left to its own devices past the harvesting stage, broccoli will sprout edible flowers, which can be served as a part of salads or as a garnish. You may have also seen multiple types of broccoli at your local farmer's market, including a variety of colors like purple and black! Created and harvested in the 1500s, broccoli has only made its appearance on American's plate in the 1700s. Kale was cultivated from the leaves of the wild mustard plant and over hundreds of years it became the curly, cabbage-like collard green we know and enjoy today. Subspecies of kale, including cavolo nero, have also developed through the process of selective breeding and it's specific nutrients within these different varieties that give them their distinctive look. Point is, these vegetables and other common vegetables have only been around for the last few hundreds of years and were never consumed prior to that. But I digress. From a single plant, over hundreds of years, we were able to cultivate dozens of new subspecies, the 6 I listed are simply the most recognizable.

Fruits

Fruit contains sugar. We have long known this to be a fact. Fructose is what gives apples, grapes, and other fruits we enjoy as part of our daily diets their characteristic sweet bite. It is so abundant that you can find pure granulated fructose at your local grocery store to be used for jam making or as a sugar replacement. While sugar itself is not inherently bad in the context of a healthy and nutritious diet in small amounts, a diet too high in sugars can lead to a myriad of health complications. Diabetes, obesity, and heart disease are at the very top of this list. The ancestral fruits of the varieties we enjoy today would, again, look very different. Early versions of blackberries would be available to gather, for instance.

Thanks again to selective breeding, we have been able to cultivate varieties of fruits, which would not only perplex our prehistoric ancestors, but would also have given them a sugar rush and surely cavities down the line. Modern fruits have been bred to have higher concentrations of sugar than their early ancestors. If you were to look at paintings from only a few centuries ago, you would see different versions of the fruits we know and love. Watermelon, for example, has been bred to have less rind and more flesh. While this makes for a delicious summertime snack, it also stands a testament to the biological innovations we, as a species, have been able to achieve.

Seedless varieties of fruits are available for purchase due to selective breeding and genetic engineering. Bananas used to be chock full of seeds before early farmers started domesticating them. As early as 7,000 years ago, bananas were cultivated in what is now Papua New Guinea and Southeast Asia. The two main varieties from which modern bananas are descended, musa acuminata and musa balbisiana, once held large hard seeds. Through the careful process of selective breeding, we now have the long (and sometimes curvy) fruit that we serve as part of a morning breakfast or as part of a decadent dessert. While bananas might be high in potassium, they are also rich in sugar. Due to the rapidly changing nature of the human diet, our food has evolved along with us and, as a result of that breeding, is a dangerously high sugar (fructose) content in some foods that we consider healthy.

What do peaches and cherries have in common? They are both fruits with a fleshy exterior and large stone in the center. While this is where most would stop at the compari-

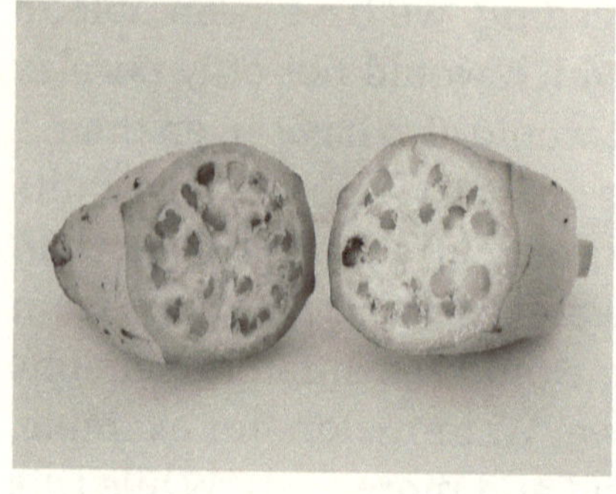

son, peaches actually used to be the size of a cherries with just a little flesh. Even as early at 4,000 B.C.E., their taste was described as "like a lentil," with an earthy taste and a hint of salt. How, then, did a cherry-sized fruit come to be the crunchy fruit we enjoy in a peach cobbler? The answer is thousands of years of selective breeding, resulting in a fruit about 64 times larger than its ancestor, with a quarter more juice and a much higher concentration of fructose.

Like we already saw, genetically modified foods may not be inherently bad itself but they do get more susceptible to disease and problems. The sugar content in some fruits, however, might have been engineered to be too high to even be considered healthy. Later on, however, we will see the kinds of issues that can arise from obsessive selective breeding.

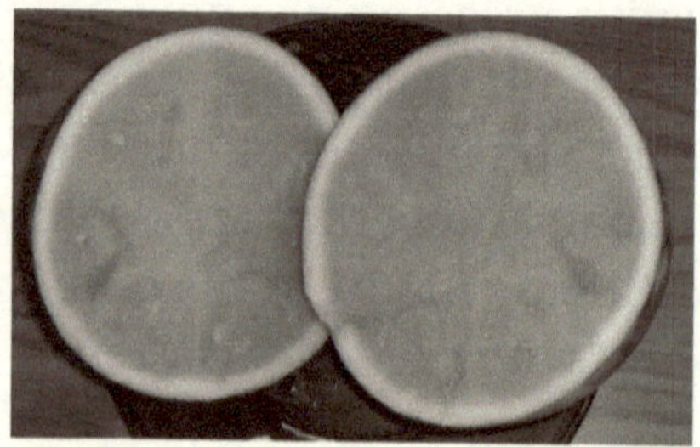

Grains

The last few years have seen the rise in gluten-free diets, which has brought into question whether or not flour is good for us in the first place. Grains are mostly comprised of carbohydrates and protein which some argue that it doesn't even need to be in the human diet. Gluten is a simple yet undigestible wheat protein that gives wheat its structure. If you were to mix together water and flour in a bowl, allow it to dry, then wash off the flour, you would be left with a lump of pure, unprocessed gluten. This is a simple science experiment you can do in the comfort of your own kitchen. For some, gluten can cause severe abdominal distress, which is why flour-based products are among the first to be cut out for elimination diets. Results may vary in elimination diets but the reason why flour is cut out is because it is known to be inflammatory.

Inflammation has a variety of causes. Injuries can cause inflammation, for instance, although in terms of diet, gluten is a known cause hence gluten intolerance. If you experience abdominal discomfort from your diet, there's a chance it could be gluten. Before you omit it completely from your diet, however, I strongly advise seeking medical advice. Modern flour is very different to what our prehistoric ancestors would have eaten. Through both evolution and selective breeding, the gluten structure has changed drastically and became a lot less tolerable for many.

Hybridization in farming is the process of interbreeding individuals of different species, or any genetically divergent plants, in order to create a new species. Our prehistoric ancestors would have started this process by cross-pollinating wild grasses, eventually resulting in einkorn wheat. The problem is with chemical hybridization, which is a relatively new concept. It only began within the last 50 years. To create wheat that is resistant to fungal disease as well as pests and to meet the demands of the industrial world, chemical hybridization was developed.

The two earliest types of wheat which we can compare to modern wheat are emmer and einkorn. You can still find emmer and einkorn flour, as well as products which are made from them. The gluten in einkorn wheat has a completely different effect on the body than modern wheat. This is due in no small part to its chromosomal structure. Einkorn is a diploid, meaning that it has just two copies of its 7 chromosomes, while modern wheat is a hexaploid, meaning that it has six copies of its chromosomes. The wheat that is used in industrial baking processes is nothing on what our prehistoric ancestors would have known.

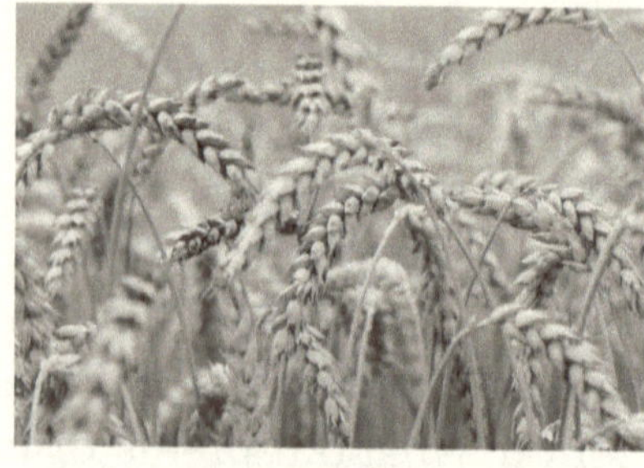

If you want to see the difference, take a handful of white flour and a handful of einkorn flour and put them on your kitchen counter. The difference between these two flours will be immediately obvious. Processed white flour, regardless of whether or not it has been bleached, is made using the endosperm (innards) of the hull. Whole einkorn flour is made using the entire hull. Modern flour is made from wheat, which was bred and processed to have a long shelf life due to the demands of industrialization. Freshly ground einkorn wheat would expire within as short as three days, due to oxidation of the small oil content. Modern wheat is refined, milled and is stripped away of its oil content and nutrients. This allows flour to have a few years on the shelf before it starts to turn. Beriberi, a thiamine (vitamin B1) deficiency, was a common disease found in rich societies in the 1800s. Only rich people could afford white bread which is why the disease was mostly prevalent in these communities. This problem was mostly resolved once we decided to enrich flour with nutrients. Nowadays it is mandatory to enrich white flour with certain nutrients, hence the term "enriched flour" when you look at nutritional facts of certain processed foods like crackers and cereals.

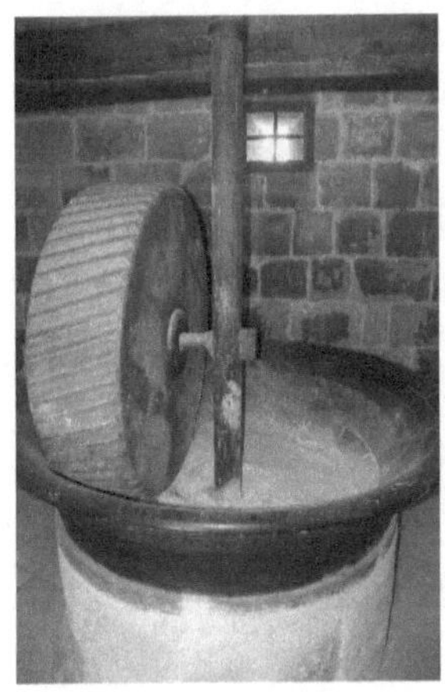

Not everyone has the ability to grow and grind their own wheat berries, hence the necessity for the bags of flour you find in the grocery store. However, if you can find a bag of unprocessed einkorn or emmer flour, I recommend finding a bread recipe which calls for it. The difference in taste, like the difference between flours, will be immediate. This isn't just the case with einkorn flour. Experiment with different grain types and starters other than conventional yeast in your bread, and other recipes than simple bread. Wheat is a dietary staple across the world so experimenting with the different varieties is key to understanding how they affect the body.

Modern Nutrition

While the abundance and variety of food we enjoy in modern times might impress our prehistoric ancestors, it is nutritionally nothing compared to what they would have enjoyed. Plants are simply not what they used to be. The process of selective breeding made it much easier for us to create new types of vegetables that we enjoy as part of a balanced diet. As a result of industrialization, our food has become less nutritional and more about the yield and shelf life. Genetic engineering has resulted in bulk quantity over quality. Although this allows for abundance, the downsides are alarming. For example, farmers who produce too much wheat are forced to burn excess crops. Industrialization has opened many opportunities while also closed many doors in the process.

As humans and our dietary needs continue to evolve, we need to ask ourselves what we actually need and whether plants in their current state are a realistic part of it. Plants are not inherently bad for us but neither are they the absolute best option. Choosing to enjoy a plant-based diet, for example, is a valid lifestyle choice, it just might not be the healthiest. Malnutrition is a common ailment often ascribed to the lack of nutritional value in vegan and vegetarian diets. On a personal level, I never felt worse than when I was vegetarian. Although I do enjoy fruits and vegetables in small quantities, I have found that a meat/animal-based diet works best for me.

Try to be more thoughtful about the fruits, vegetables, and wheat products you incorporate into your diet. While fruits and vegetables contain large amounts Vitamin C, a few minerals and calories, that may be all they provide. Oranges contain less vitamin C than they did 200 years ago. You may enjoy broccoli soup as an evening treat, but it may simply be a bowl of empty calories. This is fine on occasion, but a diet heavy in nutrient-devoid plants may end up causing more problems than benefits in the long term.

CHAPTER 2: HOW MODERN PLANTS ARE GROWN

As humans have evolved and society has progressed past industrialization, the agricultural industry has developed alongside it. Technological innovations have made it easier to sow, cultivate, and grow crops with large yields to feed the ever-growing population. This is particularly true in "first world" nations, such as the United States and United Kingdom, where 40% and 36% of the respective land is farmland. While imports add to the food source in both countries, agriculture accounts for large chunks of their respective economies. Depending on the country in question and its topography, farming techniques have evolved to incorporate new technology. One of the earliest farming techniques that has been passed down from our prehistoric ancestors to evolve alongside methods such as tilling and mechanical harvesting is now what is known as regenerative agriculture. This practice replaces monocultures with crop rotation and stops or reduces the use of chemicals and soil tilling.

Crop rotation is the practice of planting different crops in the same patch of soil to improve soil health, optimize the nutritional value of the soil, as well as combat pests and weeds. Advantages of this method include an increase in the crop yield and reduced soil erosion. Planting the same crop in the same patch of land (for example, planting nothing but corn) can lead to nutrient depletion. Once corn season is over, planting a less demanding crop in that patch of land, such as potatoes, allows the soil to recover actively. Think of it like this: if you were to spend a demanding day at the gym focusing on nothing but weight lifting, the next day you go for a light jog to keep your body active. This is a similar principle to crop rotation. Other ways soil fertility can be improved is by the biomass (roots, foliage, etc.) that is left behind. The leftover foliage decomposes and releases nutrients back into the soil and can also be eaten by livestock. Manure left behind by this livestock also improves the nutritional value of the soil for the next planting season.

While crop rotation is commonly used in farming and gardening, it can take years to perfect. This is where the disadvantages begin to show. Crops must be planted seasonally. To put it simply, crop rotation can be a gamble without the proper knowledge and resources. While it encourages crop diversification, planting the wrong crop at the wrong time or there is improper crop care can lead to diseased soil and eventual blight. Usually, this is the result of a lack of knowledge about the intricacies of crop rotation and how to properly prepare the soil for the next planting. Crop rotation requires a great amount of financial investment and, if it goes wrong, it can lead to a catastrophic harvesting season. Farmers often incur great losses early on in crop rotation due to improper implementation. Another factor which can leave crop rotation at a major disadvantage is the climate. Certain crops just won't grow in certain conditions. For example, broccoli requires a lot of sunlight while potatoes need damp conditions and minimal watering. This may sound counterproductive, but if potatoes are watered too often, it encourages fungal blight.

I realize that it sounds like I'm denouncing crop rotation when I actually don't want to sound biased. There are pros and cons to everything and this is also true when it comes to the way our food is grown. I personally believe that implementing crop rotation is the way to go, at least compared to modern monocultures. Crop rotation can be implemented anywhere but there are factors, such as the local climate, which need to be considered. Once these are addressed and worked around, appropriate measures can be taken and implemented to ensure success. Unlike monoculture farming, crop rotation offers more benefits than disadvantages. One of the ways it's beneficial is that it's much better for the environment. Practicing crop rotation results in increased carbon content in the soil. This is due to less frequent tillage in addition to less intense tillage. A result of this is that the soil gets a much-needed chance to recover from being worked so hard. Continuing along this thought, the overall structure of the soil improves. Macro pores are created, which allows for better water flow and leads to more nutrient-dense, fertile soil. This is due entirely to the increased crop residue and livestock grazing periods. While naturally-sourced pesticides and fertilizers can still be used for crop rotation, far less of them are needed than with monoculture.

Regenerative agriculture has been used for centuries, even by our prehistoric ancestors. Archaeological evidence has identified rotational fields even before history was being recorded. However, modern farming techniques may be harming our plants and subsequently our health. The only real solution is to return to the ways our early ancestors followed. That implies that we should rotate our crops, take care of our soils and use less harmful chemicals. The idea that modern farms are currently destroying the world isn't farfetched, in reality it's probably happening a lot closer to you than you think. Organic farms exist on a small scale but the ones who actually practice regenerative agriculture are even less. These are the people you find at the farmer's market, selling the crops they've grown. Later, I'll explain how buying organic produce is healthier for you. At the moment, I want you to understand that buying organic produce from a small farm is a great way to boost the local economy as well as support a practice which we sorely need to.

The Problems With Modern Growing Techniques

One of the ways in which our modern food supply is grown is through the use of monocultures. Monocultural farming is the opposite to crop rotation. It is the practice of growing a single crop in a single area. This same practice applies to livestock. While some farms may be polycultural (i.e. they grow multiple types of crops in addition to/or the use of crop rotation), they can also specialize in a particular kind of crop. However, in order to keep up with the ever-growing demand for plants, many farms have turned to monocultural farming. Unlike polycultural farming, this type of farming only has barely any benefits: it maximizes the crop yield, increases pesticide resistance, and is easier to manage. The disadvantages outweigh the advantages. As we saw with crop rotation, the soil is healthier. With so many of the same type of crop growing in the same plot of land, by the end of the growing season the soil becomes nutrient deficient.

As farmers are forced to continue monocultural practices, soil fertility will be lost, leading to potentially devastating environmental problems. Aside from this, pest control becomes much more unpredictable. While it may seem more straightforward by allowing farmers to predict pest patterns, what can actually happen is the onset of new types of pests. Grape phylloxera are insects that congregate around grapevines and are native to California. The reason I bring this up is because I want to talk about a calamitous infestation of grape phylloxera which occurred in California in the 1980s. Farmers had to uproot and replant over 2 million acres of grapevines after the plants were completely destroyed. These tiny little insects mutated over just a few short years and fed on the roots, leading to a complete economic disaster for both farmers and the California wine industry.

Moving on from the economic disaster that can befall farmers and industries, monocultures provide ample health-related problems. No matter what the crop, plants require numerous resources to grow and thrive. This comes in

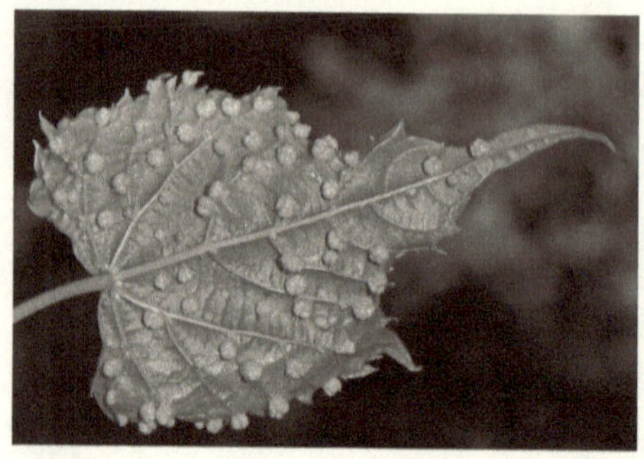

many forms: natural compost, abundant water, man-made fertilizer, chemical and natural pesticides, and a variety of financial commitments. Ultimately, this limits the plant's chances for survival. Farmers often commit to a single type of crop in order to focus their resources and maintain profits. While this is a logical and practical decision in many respects, it is not the best in terms of our health and nutrition, nor the environment. Monocultural farming leads to limited food options. Consumers such as you or I may have options through the grocery store, but think in terms of developing countries. Scarce or limited resources can lead to malnutrition. As we saw in the previous chapter, fruits and vegetables are less nutrient-dense than their prehistoric ancestors. Imagine subsisting on a single meal for a week. It could be rice, beans and bread or it could be a plate of potatoes and carrots with a little seasoning. While you would satisfy your hunger, you would quickly become malnourished.

Pollution

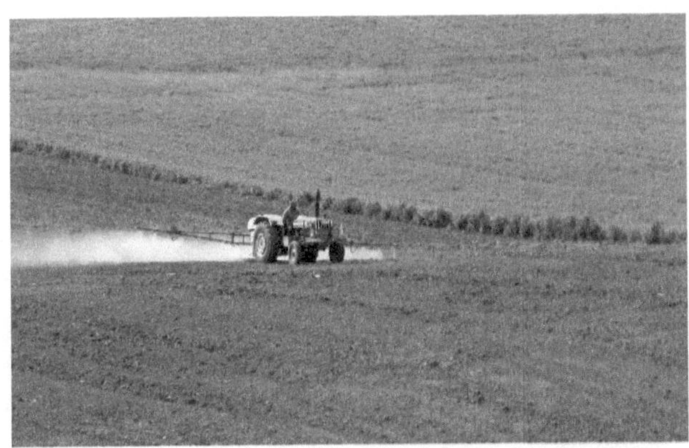

One of the biggest problems with farming on the scale that is demanded is the problem of pollution. We all understand how cars, planes, and modern technology require fossil fuels for energy, but we forget how this applies to the scale of agriculture. Tractors may require fossil fuels in order to run and you may have seen the ongoing debate regarding chemical pesticides and their effect on climate change. Fertilizers, for instance, are well-known to provide much-needed nutrition to crops in monoculture farms. This is to account for the depletion in nutrients from the growing of a single crop in a single space. Natural compost can be used as a fertilizing agent but it is often not enough, and applying too much can erode the soil and damage plant roots. An unfortunate side effect of this is that fertilizers often contaminate the local water supply. In the last five years, researchers have found alarming spikes in nitrate concentrations in communal water supplies. Rivers and lakes from which entire populations draw their water end up contaminated through chemical pollutants as a result of excessive farming.

Another way in which groundwater and water supplies can be polluted is through the use of chemical pesticides.

Soil erosion is a huge part of this transference. This was observed even in the 1980s in some of the largest US farming regions, where pesticide concentration in streams were once "very low" at a mere 5% but, as the decades have worn on and fish populations have begun to plummet, recent research indicates that the once low percentages may have increased by half to 7.5%. Research does indicate that pesticides are soluble and will degrade rapidly to "reduce their toxic effects on aquatic systems," although the hope this offers may be too slim to count on.

Tilling

When farming machinery was developed, tilling the soil solved numerous problems. It was a way to quickly prepare seedbeds, suppress weeds, aerate the soil and cover crops in a few simple steps. Tillage provided a lot of solutions and it was easy, it didn't require as much energy as it took to individually prepare each plot for seeding. Tilling also provided a means to incorporate fertilizers, such as manure, into the soil while also distributing pesticides. However, while this might have helped in the early days of modern farming, it has since come to light that tillage is perhaps the worst thing for soil.

Tillage fractures the soil, releasing carbon into the atmosphere (increasing greenhouse emissions) and compromising its quality. Not only does it disrupt the structure of the soil, it accelerates surface runoff as well as soil erosion. Surface runoff refers to the flow of water from the ground level; for example, when rain falls and it runs down an incline towards a river or it can no longer infiltrate or moisturize the soil, this is referred to as "runoff." Soil erosion is a form of soil degradation. It is the continued displacement of the upper layer of soil. While this does occur during natural phenomena such as storms, the level of damage is negligible to the amount caused by frequent tillage. Additionally, tillage reduces crop residue, which protects the soil against the force of raindrops. Without this, soil can become dislodged and broken, being "splashed" away and clog soil pores, sealing off the surface. A direct result of this is poor water infiltration, which means that crops cannot get the hydration they need to grow.

This is a problem because, as greenhouse emissions keep climbing up, our planet is slowly getting warmer and warmer. Soil, after close inspection, is a complex structure with millions of tiny creatures who all play a significant role for soil health. A healthy soil is actually carbon negative, meaning it pulls carbon from the atmosphere and buries it in the ground where it's supposed to be. Mechanical tilling destroys the soil and kills all the tiny little creatures crucial for good soil health. It removes the ability for soil to store carbon and actually releases carbon into the atmosphere, accelerating climate change.

One alternative to tilling is to use chickens. This is commonly used by smaller farms and more commonly used by hobbyist gardeners. Chickens do the same thing as tillage but on a smaller scale and not nearly to such a damaging extent. They turn over the soil and keep it nice and loose, as well as fertilizing it with their manure as they go about digging up potential pests. Another method is to add a little compost. This enriches the soil with vital nutrients in addition to keeping it nice and loose. This also improves soil structure, reducing erosion.

As tillage continue over many seasons and, subsequently, many years, the impact becomes more devastating. The complete and utter breakdown of soil quality is assured. While there are methods to prevent this from happening, they are short term at best. Root elongation is what helps plants grow and take in the nutrients they need from the soil. Broken soil does contain nutrients, but, as the years go on, we will continue to see soil infertility become an increasing issue. Additionally, the structure is often so eroded that plant roots cannot break through it. It would not be unexpected if, in the near future, the farming industry was forced to do a complete overhaul in order to address this.

Dead Zones

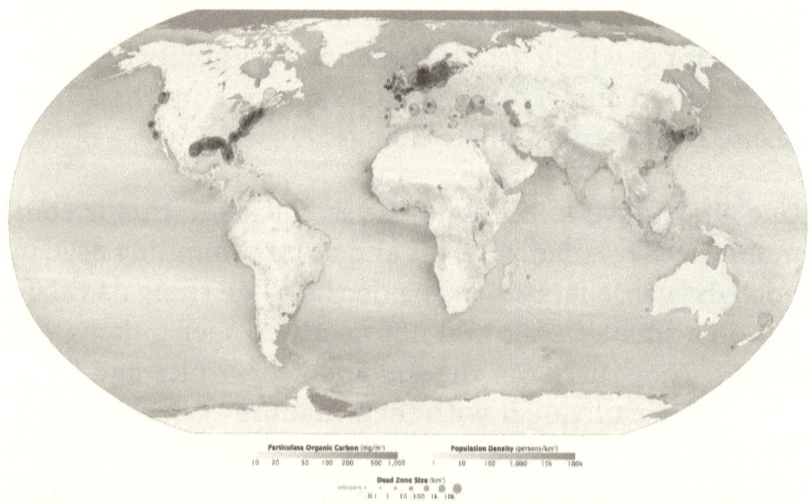

Dead zones have been gaining attention in the scientific

community lately. Large pockets of the oceans, as well as smaller bodies of water like rivers and lakes, become so devoid of oxygen that it is impossible for any aquatic life to thrive. For this reason, they abandon it and that part of the ocean is declared a 'dead zone.' Dead zones are a thing because of eutrophication, which happens when a body of water, such as a lake or a river, is too full of nutrients. These nutrients are most commonly phosphorus and nitrogen based, both of which are extremely toxic in large amounts and can be catastrophic.

Remember when we talked about agricultural runoffs? Ocean dead zones are directly correlated with agricultural runoffs. The increased intensity of agricultural practices, together with a rapidly growing population, as well as industrial activity, has led to a significant rise in eutrophication. Massive amounts of phosphorus and nitrogen and other chemicals found in herbicides and pesticides are being emitted as a result of these key factors. The scale is difficult to imagine but these two nutrients, which might be vital for plants, are a detriment to aquatic ecosystems. They enter the air, soil, and water. Although different regions emit different levels of these two nutrients, larger nations such as the United States are heavily reliant on commercial fertilizers and animal manure. Both of these are present in monoculture farming. All of the world's water supplies are connected and while it might seem like a stretch to think that the runoff from a farm in Michigan can have an effect on the Pacific Ocean, this is exactly what happens. Eutrophication has increased because of this exact process. This also happens as a result of untreated wastewaters in developing countries. While sewage treatment is an important part of maintaining a hygienic society, these facilities are less regulated in some parts or the world, where waste is dumped into local bodies of water such as creeks, lakes, or rivers.

The Solution?

Returning to the start of this chapter, regenerative agriculture is the solution to our modern problems caused by bad agricultural practices. Monocultures, pesticide/chemicals overuse and soil tilling, all contribute to environmental destruction. While regenerative agriculture is in practice in some parts of the world, it is viewed as more economically viable to commit to monocultures. Soil tilling contributes enormously to earths harming temperatures and can only be resolved if we treat our soils correctly. The benefits of crop rotation outweigh the downsides, which all amount to the knowledge and practice it takes to perfect. Combined with a less frequent use of chemical pesticides and more emphasis on organic, naturally-source pesticides and fertilizers, the solution to the problem of modern farming techniques is to make it more economically viable. Although there are changes underway to meet this end, this is still years away. Right now, if you would like to take advantage of polycultural and organic produce, a solution is to visit your local farmer's market or to grow your own. We will cover these in more detail later on.

CHAPTER 3: THE PROBLEM WITH PLANT-BASED NUTRITION

Food is something to be enjoyed as well as fuel for your body, and having plants as part of a diet can add some flavor and variety. In order to get the most out of the food we eat, our diets have to be balanced. A balanced diet can include a wide variety of foods, both "healthy" and "unhealthy." One of the purported benefits of the vegetarian and vegan diets is that they are "healthier" due to the wider variety of nutritional sources. However, nutritional facts are not set in stone and are far from a fact. Although it might say on google or chronometer that there's vitamin A in spinach it is not the case. Vegetarians and vegans who do not aim for variety experience iron deficiency, anemia, and vitamin deficiencies. These are also concerns for anyone who aims to be more plant-based. Plant-based diets are nutritionally devoid of certain essential vitamins, minerals and amino acids only found in meats and dairy products.

The vegetarian diet actually has the benefit of being supplemented by dairy products. These provide essential fats and proteins which cannot be found in a purely plant-based diet. However, most vegetarians take over the counter supplements to account for minerals and vitamins lost. While there are many sources of plant-based protein, this is still something many vegetarians struggle to include in their diet, and some of the sources have negative effects. Mycoprotein, for example, is derived from mushrooms. Side effects can include vomiting, nausea, and diarrhea. There have even been cases of allergic reactions to mycoprotein. Most vitamin supplements out there in the market are synthetic, which means they're created in a lab. Since they are not the real thing, your body will have a difficult time trying to absorb them and using it.

The best known source of protein for both the vegan and vegetarian diets is soy. In order to be turned into soy milk, soy cheese, and soy yogurt, soya beans have to be turned into soy isolate protein powder. Soy protein comes with its benefits. It's low calorie, low fat, low in carbohydrates, and, depending on the form it takes, it can be high in fiber. People who suffer from dairy allergies use soy products to replace milks, cheeses, and even butters. Vegans, vegetarians and allergy sufferers alike praise soy as a nutritional powerhouse. As I mentioned, soy protein does have its benefits but it's far from a nutritional powerhouse. Soy intolerance have been known to develop in people after overconsuming soy for years.

In this chapter, I am going to introduce you to the essential nutrients missing in a plant-based diet. I'm also going to explain how plants are marketed to seem "more nutritionally dense" than a diet which includes meat. Vitamins, minerals, amino acids, etc., play a key role in keeping your body up and functioning. The best way to obtain these nutrients is from eating high quality animal foods. High quality meaning grass-fed cattle, pasture raised animals, wild caught fish, unpasteurized dairy and raw cheeses. Nutrients from animal products are more readily bioavailable to the human body than nutrients from plant foods.

Essential Vitamins And Minerals

I want to use this next section to explore some of the more vital minerals and vitamins. One of the biggest misunderstanding about nutrition is that "you are what you absorb". Though this proverb isn't entirely false, it is much more accurate to say "you are what you absorb". You see, not all vitamins, minerals and elements are absorbed once you eat them. There are multiple types and variations of vitamins and minerals. Usually, the variations are apparent once you compare, let's say, vitamin A from a plant source or a food that comes from animal origin. It's a war against plant nutrition and animal nutrition. Unfortunately for plant-based dieters, omnivores and people who eat meat will win. Animal versions of vitamins and minerals are much more bioavailable than plant versions. Bioavailable simply means it is more accessible or better absorbed by the human body.

If you go to your local grocery store, you will find supplements and multivitamins, which you might purchase to help you achieve your recommended daily intake of each vitamin and mineral. While some might brush these off as a way to produce "overpriced urine," they can actually be essential for people who suffer from certain deficiencies. Supplemental iron tablets and powders, for example, can be helpful to people who struggle with iron deficiency anemia. If you want to prepare your immune system for flu season, taking real Vitamin C tablets for about six weeks before flu season begins is an effective way to safeguard you against seasonal illnesses. What I'm saying is that supplements have their benefits. The body gets rid of what it doesn't need through the renal system so you don't have much to worry about ingesting too much as long as you follow the guidelines on the bottle or instructions given to you by a medical professional. But I strongly recommend trying to get your vitamins and minerals from food, especially animal sources, like cheese, eggs or meat. The reason I say this is because, usually, supplements are synthetic and are not as effective as getting nutrients directly from food.

Retinol vs Beta-carotene (Vitamin A)

Both retinol and beta-carotene are important for the body. Without getting too much into details, retinol is the form of vitamin A that is found and used in animals. Beta-carotene, on the other hand, is the plant version of vitamin A. So, what's the difference you might ask. Well retinol is the active form of vitamin A which humans use while beta-carotene is mostly considered and antioxidants. Lucky for us, beta-carotene can be converted to retinol through the digestive process. In order for this to happen, you need a healthy intestinal tract, sufficient biles salts from a healthy gallbladder, and specific enzymes.

You probably know Vitamin A from the WW2-era propaganda campaign where a British pilot attributed his keen eyesight to eating plenty of carrots. Though he might have had good eyesight, it surely wasn't because of the carrots he was consuming. Vitamin A is essential for a lot of functions in the body. Eyesight is only one of the functions it supports. It occurs naturally in eggs and liver.

Synthetic versions of vitamin A are also available over the counter or via prescription in varying strengths. It is used in skincare products and as a dietary supplement, depending on how it is synthesized. Among the downsides, using it can cause irritation and redness in new users, and it isn't absorbed as effectively as naturally-sourced Vitamin A. Accutane is a popular synthetic vitamin A that is currently sold as an acne treatment, but it can have major side-effects, such as liver damage.

In order to properly convert beta-carotene into retinol, you need the BCM01 gene. Healthy adults typically convert about ⅙ of beta-carotene into usable Vitamin A, while infants are unable to. Assuming that your digestive tract is healthy and you eat plenty of plants which are purported to be "high" in beta-carotene, in order to produce a single unit of retinol, you would need six units of beta-carotene. When taken in as part of a healthy diet, beta-carotene is better absorbed with fats. This is why we need bile salts for the conversion to be possible: bile breaks down fats and the beta-carotene along with it.

Vitamin D3

Also known as cholecalciferol, there are many sources of Vitamin D3. While it is present in some food, the best way to get ahold of it is from sitting in front of the sun as it can be absorbed from ultraviolet (UVB) rays. Once hit by the sun's rays, dehydrocholesterol (a type of cholesterol) reacts with it to start vitamin D3 synthesis. However, it is biologically inert and must undergo hydroxylation. The first hydroxylation happens through the liver, where it is converted into calcifediol. The second hydroxylation occurs in the kidneys, where it is converted into calcitriol, the active form of Vitamin D. This process also occurs when taking Vitamin D from food or supplements. There's also a plant version of vitamin D called vitamin D2. This version is known to not be as efficient as vitamin D3.

Because Vitamin D3 can be absorbed from UV rays, deficiency and inadequate levels has a seasonal stimulus. It has been recorded that Vitamin D3 also plays a vital role in maintaining a healthy immune system. A study in 2018 showed that "a significant effect is also the suppression of inflammatory processes." These occur in cases of infection, sudden raise in temperature, or injury. Seasonal flu, for example, is an inflammatory process. The role of Vitamin D3 in preventing flu infection is still being investigated but, for now, it can be prescribed as a treatment.

Vitamin D3 is essential for calcium absorption, which is why some dairy brands sell milk and cheese which have been fortified with extra Vitamin D3. In order to maintain healthy serum calcium and phosphate levels for bone mineralization, it needs to be a huge part of your diet. This vitamin is also essential for bone shaping and remodeling, for example if you break a bone. In recent years, the United States and Canada have seen a rise in Vitamin D3 deficiency.

Cholecalciferol (vitamin D3) is also known as a steroid hormone which is derived from cholesterol. Vitamin D3 deficiency is common in people who follow a low cholesterol diet or dairy free diet. Vitamin D3 deficiency is common in people who follow a dairy free diet. A deficiency of Vitamin D3 can lead to hypocalcemic tetany (an involuntary contraction of muscles). Insufficient Vitamin D3 can lead to rickets in children and osteomalacia in adults. Rickets is a disease which primarily affects children; it causes soft, weak, and brittle bones, which can lead to skeletal deformities such as bowed legs. An adult version of rickets is known as osteomalacia, which causes soft bones and can lead to fractures. Both of these conditions can be solved with an increased intake of Vitamin D3. This can be done through more sun exposure, in the form of a dietary change or through over the counter or prescription supplements. Light panels simulating the sun's rays or tanning beds might also be a good solution.

Vitamin B12

Vitamin B_{12} is one of the multiple B vitamins. Though there are only 8 popular ones, some say there could be as many as hundreds of B vitamins. This vitamin is heavily involved in the body's metabolic processes, including cell metabolism,

DNA synthesis, and in fatty acid and amino acid metabolism. It's also known as cobalamin and helps with the creation and health of red blood cells.

While all vitamins and minerals are important for nutrition, you can probably guess that B12 is the one you absolutely need. Too little B12 in your diet can lead to Vitamin B12 deficiency anemia (lack of red blood cells). Symptoms of regular anemia include fatigue, lethargy, breathlessness, lightheadedness, heart palpitations, tinnitus, a loss of appetite, and sudden or rapid weight loss. In addition to these, Vitamin B12 deficiency anemia symptoms include: glossitis (sore, red tongue), mouth ulcers, a yellow tinge to the skin, irritability, depression, decline in cognitive functioning (such as memory loss and impaired judgement), and paraesthesia (pins and needles).

Plant-based diets, in particular the vegan diet, is completely devoid of naturally occurring B12. In order to get a decent amount, you would have to take over the counter B12 supplements as the only sources of B12 are animal-based. These sources include fish, certain cheeses, meat, milk, and eggs. You can even find "fortified" breakfast cereals, which contain increased levels of B12. Keep in mind that fortified foods are usually fortified with synthetic vitamins, not the real thing. Which means that it is potentially less efficient compared to real vitamins. It is true that B12 producing bacteria live in dirt and on plants. But consuming these bacteria hasn't been shown to populate the gut nor to even survive stomach acid. Maybe a fecal microbiota transplant could help.

Vitamin B12 is only absorbed in the last part of the small intestine, the ileum. Since B12 is bound to animal proteins and gastric acid, pepsin needs to break down the proteins in order for B12 to be released. However, gut wall problems can interrupt its absorption into the body. Even in people who eat a balanced diet, gut problems can be enough to cause B12 deficiency anemia. Individual therapeutic approaches can help resolve B12 malabsorption, although it needs to be handled on a case-by-case basis.

Vitamin K2

Vitamin K2 is probably the most overlooked vitamin out there. Not a lot of people know it exist, yet it might be the most important one. In general, Vitamin K is a fat-soluble vitamin best known for the role it plays in blood clotting. However, there are several different K Vitamins and they all serve different roles. The best known variants of Vitamin K are Vitamin K1 and Vitamin K2. Vitamin K1 is responsible for blood coagulation. For example, if you suffer a dermal abrasion (scarring), the blood coagulates and forms a scab. On the other hand, Vitamin K2 plays a central role in the metabolization of calcium. K2 is known to work with D3 to absorb and place calcium in appropriate areas, like bones and teeth. Vitamin K1 is found mostly in leafy green vegetables such as spinach, kale, and collard greens. Animal products, such as raw cheeses, egg yolks and fermented foods are the best sources of Vitamin K2. Your gut can also produce Vitamin K2. Structurally, both vitamins are very different. Vitamin K1 has a shorter chain and is only present in the body for a few hours, whereas Vitamin K2 has a longer chain and is present in the body for up to two days after ingestion.

To make things more complicated than they already are, there are multiple versions of Vitamin K2, including MK-4, MK-7, MK-9 and others. While they might seem like cool assault rifle names, there are a few slight differences between an assault rifle and a vitamin, but I digress. Vitamin K1 can be converted into K2 but only in the form of MK-4, which leaves you with the other forms of K2 missing.

A deficiency of Vitamin K2 is more common than a Vitamin K1 deficiency, which is almost nonexistent. Symptoms of Vitamin K2 deficiency include easy bruising, secretions from nose and mouth, excessive bleeding from wounds, heavy menstruation in women, blood in the urine or stool, and bleeding from the gastrointestinal tract. This deficiency has multiple causes. The first, and easiest to correct, is diet. Simply add a few Vitamin K2-rich foods into your diet, possibly with a supplement, and it will correct itself. A second cause is through certain medications. For example, the anticoagulant medication warfarin or certain antibiotics. Since antibiotics target bacteria, this can prevent the gut from producing its own bacteria which can manufacture Vitamin K2. If you are in need of or taking either of these medications, consult your doctor if you're concerned about possible Vitamin K2 deficiency. Another cause is fat malabsorption, which is a metabolic disorder that prevents fat from being absorbed. This most commonly occurs in people who struggle with celiac disease or cystic fibrosis.

The treatment for a general Vitamin K deficiency, in most cases, is the drug phytonadione, also known as Vitamin K1. It can be prescribed as an oral medication, but if you are taking an anticoagulant, chances are you will be given a smaller dose than a patient who is not taking an anticoagulant. Because there is no set or minimum amount of Vitamin K which you should eat every day, the best course of action to prevent a deficiency is to ensure that you are eating a balanced diet with plenty of sources of K vitamins.

Vitamin B6

Pyridoxine, also known as Vitamin B6, is a water-soluble vitamin which the body needs for several key roles.

Vitamin B6 is found in plant foods but pyridoxal 5-phosphate, the active form of B6, is mostly found in animal foods and tends to have a decreased presence in plant foods. Pyridoxal, pyridoxamine, and pyridoxal are the inactive forms that are prevalent in plant foods, which are less bioavailable. You need to have the enzyme pyridoxal 5-phosphate synthase to convert inactive forms into the active form. The active form has a huge role in protein, fat, and carbohydrate metabolism. It also assists in the creation of neurotransmitters. Since the active form of B6 is used in the metabolism process of protein, fats, and carbohydrates, it is a fair assumption that having a lack of the active form in your diet will make it harder to gain muscle and get energy.

DHA and EPA

Eicosapentaenoic acid (EPA) and docosahexaenoic acid (DHA) are an essential part of a proper diet. DHA and EPA are fatty acids commonly known as omega 3 oils. Omega 3 oils are good for brain functions as well as the blood.

Without Omega-3 fatty acids, our blood cells would not have strong cell membranes. They are found in animal products, most notably fish. Over the counter supplements are often advertised as "omega 3 fish oil" for this reason. However, I still recommend getting DHA and EPA from natural sources rather than supplements because the omega 3 in supplements might be old and oxidized. DHA and EPA have also been shown to have a role in the health of the heart. Triglycerides are a type of fat which can build up in the bloodstream. Having elevated levels of triglycerides puts patients at a high risk of heart disease, however omega 3 oils like DHA and EPA can help lower high levels of triglycerides.

As mentioned earlier, EPA and DHA are typically found in animal. ALA (Alpha Linolenic Acid), on the other hand, is the omega 3 found in plant sources. Our bodies can only utilize DHA and EPA leaving ALA at the third place on the podium. Your body can convert ALA into EPA and DHA if it needs to, but only in a very small amount. So low in fact that you cannot rely purely on ALA to get the animal version (active form) of omega 3 (EPA and DHA). The conversion rate is even lower when your diet is high in omega 6 (Alpha-Linoleic Acid).

There are multiple types of fat which we need in our diet and the one I am currently mentioning is classified as a polyunsaturated fat. The body takes longer to break them down because they have a more complex structure than monounsaturated fat. A deficiency of omega-3 fatty acids can lead to a variety of health complications. One of the early signs of omega-3 deficiency is dry, easily irritated skin. Studies have shown that taking supplements rich in omega-3 fatty acids can improve the integrity of skin cells, which leads to improved skin health. Another common sign of deficiency is joint pain. Omega-3 fatty acids play an important role in joint health. It's normal for the body to get stiff and achy as it ages but a diet deficient in omega-3 fatty acids, such as DHA and EPA, can cause this to happen much sooner. Eating foods which are rich in omega-3 fatty acids and taking high quality supplements can help to improve joint health.

Nonheme Iron vs Heme Iron

Iron is an important mineral that our bodies need to produce rich, healthy blood. There are two kinds of iron which are currently available in our diets: heme iron and nonheme iron. Heme iron comes from animal foods, such as meat and fish. As its name suggests, heme iron comes from hemoglobin and proteins which are found in meats. Nonheme iron is found in leafy green vegetables such as spinach, grains like wheat, and pulses such as beans. Both kinds of iron are bioavailable to us but heme iron is much more common and easier for the body to absorb. In 2010, a study suggested that mixed diets (consisting of a mix of animal and plant foods) have an iron bioavailability of 14-18%, while plant-based diets (consisting of only plant foods, potentially with some dairy products for vegetarians) have an iron bioavailability of 5-12%. In 2020, a study suggested that iron absorption can be improved by taking supplements on alternate days.

The most common symptom of iron deficiency is iron deficiency anemia. Iron deficiency anemia is a medical condition where the blood lacks healthy red blood cells. Iron, both heme and nonheme, are important in the production of hemoglobin, which allows the blood to carry oxygen. This condition is characterized by extreme fatigue, sudden weight loss, shortness of breath, fast heartbeat, cold hands and feet, brittle nails, and pale skin. Iron deficiency anemia is most common in a vegan diet, where heme iron is absent from the diet. Iron deficiency anemia can be treated with iron supplementation in the form of a shot or a supplement pill. However, the best way to treat it is through preventative action, such as eating a diet rich in bioavailable heme iron.

Another common iron-related ailment which tends to go unnoticed is iron toxicity, also known as iron poisoning. Even though our bodies need iron, taking too much in the form of an over the counter supplement or fortified wheat can cause significant repercussions to our health and wellbeing. There are two common manifestations of iron toxicity: corrosive or cellular. Corrosive iron toxicity causes damage to the gastrointestinal mucosa (such as the stomach or intestinal linings), which results in nausea, vomiting, abdominal pain, and diarrhea. On a cellular level, it can cause impairments to the cellular metabolism of the heart, liver, and central nervous system. This occurs when free iron collects and concentrates in the mitochondria, inhibiting specific functions, such as oxidative phosphorylation, which are needed to power the cells. This ultimately leads to the death of the cell.

Symptoms of iron poisoning include seizures, dizziness, weak pulse, low blood pressure, fever, pulmonary embolism (fluid in the lungs), jaundice, and headaches. These are the early symptoms, although more serious complications such as liver failure can occur if iron toxicity is left untreated. Deferoxamina, also known as desferal, is currently being used to treat iron toxicity. It works by binding free iron and chelating a complex structure that cannot be unbound and absorbed into the bloodstream; this is then excreted through the renal (kidney, urinary) system. If the levels of toxicity are too great, dialysis may be implemented.

Cholesterol

Cholesterol is a carrier for triglycerides as well as for other nutrients and elements. Your body makes around 3,000 mg every day which represents around 75% of all the cholesterol in your body, meaning the 25% left needs to come from diet. 10% of all cholesterol produced is made in the brain. There are two key types of cholesterol: low-density lipoprotein (LDL, the so called "bad" cholesterol) and high-density lipoprotein (HDL, the so called "good" cholesterol). Broadly speaking, cholesterol is the waxy substance found in your blood and every cell in your body. Some cholesterol is necessary to keep our cells and organs healthy. The liver is capable of producing all the cholesterol the body needs, although it can be found in foods such as meat, eggs, poultry, and some dairy products.

There's a lot of controversy surrounding cholesterol being the cause of heart disease. The lipid hypothesis, suggest that the higher your LDL level is, the higher your risk for cardiovascular heart disease among other serious conditions. Without getting too deep into it, the lipid hypothesis has been debunked multiple times now. If you have blood-work on hand, true markers for heart disease risk are if your HDL is to low contrasted with too high triglycerides, LDL is not a marker for anything. For more information on this, I recommend edifying yourself on Dave Feldman's work.

If your triglycerides are too high and HDL too low, you can be put at risk of heart disease among other serious conditions. This is because overconsumption of inflammatory foods can lead to the build-up of plaque, which is a fatty substance that narrows the arteries and prevents the blood from circulating. This is the leading cause of a heart attack. However, blocked blood flow can also cause a stroke, which occurs when blood flow to the brain is blocked. In modern times, it is very easy to come accross and consume inflammatory foods that can damage your body and deplete you from nutrients. A lot of vegan food is highly processed in order to replicate the shape and texture of the meat product it is designed to replace, which is way worse than just eating a steak. In addition, a lot of cooking oils used in vegan cooking are not as heart healthy as people might think. Canola oil, for example, has gotten an amazing reputation as being heart healthy but it is very far from the truth. It is very inflammatory for the body as it contains loads of oxidized omega 6.

Point is cholesterol is a nutrient critical for good human health and development. It mostly serves as a precursor for steroid hormone synthesis. Steroid hormones mostly include sex hormones, which are estrogen and testosterone. A diet too low in cholesterol might put you at a risk of hormone imbalance or deficiency. For teens, this might slow down their growing rate as well as cause late puberty.

Heart Disease - A Case

Since the 1960s, it has been concluded, mostly by Ancel Keys and his team, that saturated fat and cholesterol was the cause of CHD. However, in recent years, we have seen a surge of studies that have questioned the wisdom of this course of action. The current model is to set targets in the reduction of LDL cholesterol, but a study which took place between 2018-20 identified that other factors might be at play. As we saw above, deficiencies in certain vitamins and minerals can significantly affect the heart. One of the more practical factors in this is the amount of stress on the individual. Cortisol, also known as the "stress hormone," together with adrenaline, can thicken the blood, which lowers blood pressure and restricts blood flow. This can deplete the body of nutrients. It's also no coincidence that heart attacks occur after a period of stress. This causes changes to your blood that contribute to the build-up of arterial plaque. The initial cause for plaque buildup is usually caused by a small fissure in the arterial wall. The body tries to heal the area by sticking somewhat of a homemade bandaid on it, known as a plaque. Fissures usually occur because of a Vitamin C deficiency, it's like a form of scurvy.

Cholesterol plays a vital role in cellular repair, so targeting it might not be the best course of action. Instead, another course of action might be to examine mineral and vitamin deficiencies. We've already talked about how iron toxicity can lead to cellular death. Another factor that was recently identified is Vitamin D deficiency. As we have already covered, the classic function Vitamin D is the gastrointestinal absorption of calcium. Observational studies as early as the 1980s have suggested an indirect link between Vitamin D and cardiovascular health. More recently, between 2000-2004, the link was further studied and, although it has not yet been made clear, we can understand that Vitamin D plays a vital role in cardiovascular health. One of the proposed theories is that it plays a preventative role in inflammation. At the time of writing this, studies are still ongoing.

Heart disease is a very complex problem, which is still to this day the leading cause of death in the US and second for Canada. It's really sad to say but drug sellers and pharmaceutical companies make a lot of money off of people being sick. Unfortunately, the cure for a lot of modern diseases has all been found a long time ago but it keeps getting brush under the carpep, ignored or deliberately hidden from us. The reason for this is because healthy people do not generate money for a lot of companies, including hospitals, pharmaceutical companies and drug manufacturers. If you want to reduce your risk of CHD, avoid inflammatory foods like vegetable oils, sugar and refined products. Include lots of foods rich in amino acids, vitamin K2 and vitamin C in your diet.

A new observational study from May 28 2020 suggests that a higher vitamin K2 intake will lower the risk for CHD. As we saw earlier, vitamin K2 is necessary to properly transport calcium where it belongs, in the bones. It is no surprise that consuming more vitamin K2 produces this type of result. The study also mentions that vitamin K1 (plant version) intake did not produce the same beneficial effect.

Conclusion

The essential vitamins and minerals we need in our diet are easy enough to come by through balanced nutrition including a variety of animal food products. However, as we have seen, a nutritionally unbalanced diet can cause significant health problems. Iron toxicity, for example, is less well-known than iron deficiency anemia. All of the health problems I listed can be treated with preventative action, such as a balanced diet. In the case of heart disease, scientists and health professionals are learning more every day about the link between vitamin deficiencies and the onset of heart problems. It is becoming clearer every day that LDL cholesterol might not be the culprit. Following a diet which is devoid of essential minerals and vitamins leaves your health at a detriment. While the body has processes such as excretion to eliminate all waste resources, these cannot be relied upon. Taking care of your body is a difficult task and a great way to start is through proper nutrition with lots of bioavailable nutrients from animal sources.

Speaking of a proper nutrition, in the next section, we are going to cover a less talked about type of "nutrient," the antinutrient.

CHAPTER 4:
ANTINUTRIENTS

A nutrient is a substance which is necessary for growth and development. The body depends on getting nutrients from a proper diet to maintain important functions. Vegetables do contain nutrients, just not as many as are marketed. As we saw in the previous section, plant-based diets are lacking in many essential minerals and vitamins. While supplements can be added to improve your uptake rate, it is possible that a plant-based diet is doing more nutritional harm than good.

It's time to explore the antinutrient.

Getting To Know Antinutrients

Just like sugar is present in everything we eat, antinutrients are present in all plant foods. They can be denatured and degraded through a variety of modern cooking methods, but even once the plants have been cooked, the antinutrients remain. One common carrier of the antinutrient is seeds. Think of the roasted pumpkin seeds you might find in the snack aisle at the grocery store. These seeds have been bred and prepared in order to provide minimal nutritional value while also remaining sterile; once they pass through your digestive tract, they will no longer be viable for sprouting new crops. However, if you were to go to a whole foods store or prepare the same pumpkin seeds from a freshly-grown pumpkin, the story changes. The seeds from a fresh pumpkin are still fertile, which is why farmers and gardeners might keep them for the next growing season. When they leave your digestive tract, they have been broken down and can grow into a new plant.

To put it simply, seeds are designed to be eaten and go right through the gut, and this includes animals and humans. They bind to minerals during digestion. When excreted, they are basically stealing nutrients. This process happens to give the seedlings an extra boost to ensure proper growth. In the next section, we are going to look at some common antinutrients and how they affect the human body.

What Are Antinutrients?

An antinutrient is a compound found in plants and plant-based food, which inhibits the absorption of essential minerals and nutrients. Societies that base their diets on grains and legumes are particularly at risk of malnutrition from antinutrients since these are the two plant groups where antinutrients are more prevalent. Corn, for example, is nutritionally void unless it has gone through a process called nixtamalization. This process changes the pH level and loosens the cellulose, making it easier to digest.

Antinutrients are common in plant-based diets. They are not inherently "bad" but they can cause problems if over-consumed. While they may not be an issue for those who enjoy a balanced diet, anyone who eats a purely plant-based diet is at risk of malnutrition from antinutrients.

These nasty compounds not only steal nutrients from you but can also severely damage your gut lining. This may not alert a lot of people, but gut damage is a serious problem. It starts with malabsorption, skin issues, leaky gut and can lead to terrible autoimmune conditions, such as eczema, dermatitis, Crohn's disease and more. Most people don't know this, but autoimmune conditions can get resolved. Removing antinutrients from the diet will dramatically improve these conditions.

Common Antinutrients

Antinutrients are present in all plant foods and, just like the varieties of plants you can eat, there are numerous types of antinutrients. There are too many to list in this book, so I encourage you to learn more about them. Below, I'm going to list and explain the most commonly found antinutrients in plant foods.

- **Phytate (phytic acid):** In plants, the role of phytate is to store phosphorus in the plant's tissue. It forms chemical bonds with metals and proteins, which can limit the bioavailability of certain minerals and vitamins during digestion. This antinutrient is found primarily in seeds and legumes, where its content is highly varied. Beans contain anywhere from 0.6%-2.4%, whereas wheat can contain anywhere from 0.4% to 1.4%. Oats and almonds are also commonly known as "health foods" but still are crowded with antinutrients. When digested, phytate inhibits the absorption of zinc, calcium, magnesium, and iron. It does have a few benefits, including the degradation of kidney stones, and some research is being done into its anticarcinogenic effects although, at the time of writing, this information is limited and speculative at best.

- **Tannins:** These antinutrients are water-soluble polyphenols that are present in multiple plant foods. Tannins are a class of astringents due to their bitter and acidic taste. They bind to and precipitate proteins and other compounds (such as amino acids). Most commonly found in wine, tannins have a mix of effects on the human body. For example, they can accelerate blood clotting and lower blood pressure. Due to their chemical structure, tannins are considered antimicrobial, which can mean disaster for your gastrointestinal flora. The gut contains bacteria that helps break down food during digestion and these bacteria can be inhibited by tannins. But tannins are one of the lesser damaging antinutrient.

- **Lectins:** Probably the worse one out there, lectins are a class of antinutrients found in all plant foods but are most prominent in grains, legumes, and seeds. They are a protein that bonds to certain carbohydrates and inhibits the uptake of certain minerals. In their active state, they have a variety of negative side effects. For example, they can inhibit the absorption of calcium and iron. Although there has been limited research into the nature of lectins on the body, a common theme in animal and plant cell studies indicates their role in malabsorption. Lectins also play an inflammatory role and can make conditions such as rheumatoid arthritis and type 1 diabetes much worse. This is because lectins have a "staying power" when they bind to cells, meaning that the bonds they form last longer than any other bond formed by antinutrients. One of the more alarming problems this can cause is the deterioration of the gut and the eventual development of autoimmune diseases such as arthritis, eczema and more. Once your gut is damage, it because more permeable, meaning more things can go through your gut wall including things you don't want, which then triggers autoimmune responses. To put it simply, if your gut wall is too damaged, autoimmune conditions will make their appearance.

- **Calcium Oxalate:** As the name implies, calcium oxalate binds to calcium and prevents it from being absorbed. Oxalates are found in leafy green vegetables and, when it binds with calcium, it prevents calcium your body from using it. One of the most common problems with calcium oxalate is the effect it has on the renal tract, most notably in crystal form. Crystals of calcium oxalate are most commonly found in kidney stones, which themselves are just clumps of minerals that could not be absorbed.

- **Protease Inhibitors:** Protease is an enzyme which is essential for the breakdown of dietary proteins. Red meat, for example, will be broken down by protease. Seeds, legumes, and grains are particularly rich in protease inhibitors. Certain fruits, including bananas and apples, contain protease inhibitors. This particular antinutrient has been of scientific interest since the 1980s and, for a while, they were considered "nutritionally insignificant." However, a diet that is high in protein inhibitors can lead to a lot of problems. Protease inhibitors work by blocking cell growth, which can stunt repair. As a result, muscle repair will take longer after injury.

What Is The Role Of Antinutrients?

When sprouting, crop plants develop antinutrients as a deterrent from pests and herbivores. In this way, we can view antinutrients as a defense mechanism. For seeds, antinutrients has the role to capture as many minerals as it can through the animal's digestive system. Once it's out, it can freely grow with the added bonus of more minerals to ensure growth. Some modern cultivars have their antinutrients selectively bred out, although this is not the case for all of the plants we eat. The cultivars which had their antinutrients bred out are typically used as cheap feed for livestock. A great deal of research is being done into whether or not there are any benefits to antinutrients in the human body. Protease inhibitors, as we saw, can stunt cell growth. For this reason, medical protease inhibitors are currently being used as an antiretroviral drug. While this sort of research is still ongoing, it is best to limit them where we can and focus on building a diet heavy in nutrient-dense foods.

Why Are Antinutrients A Problem?

In simple terms, antinutrients play a pivotal role in inhibiting the absorption of essential minerals and nutrients. While eating plants is not itself a bad thing, eating only plants can lead to a build-up of the above antinutrients in your system. Lectins are the most prominent antinutrient and, as they inhibit iron absorption, any iron you may have taken from your food (be it heme iron or nonheme iron) is at risk of not being absorbed. This may not be a problem in the short term, since medical intervention and a few dietary changes can reverse most problems caused by antinutrients. However, in the long term, significant ailments like autoimmune diseases can be difficult to treat. Gut damage happens over years of consuming too many antinutrient containing foods. The link between gut problems and certain antinutrients has been studied in recent years and we know enough to be able to take preventative actions.

How Can I Reduce Antinutrients In My Diet?

There are a variety of methods you can implement in order to reduce the number of antinutrients in your diet. We are going to go into more detail in Chapter 7 but, for now, I can offer a couple of easy, quick fixes you can try to get yourself into the habit of reducing antinutrients in your food. First, you can boil your plants. Red beans like kidney beans contain large amounts of phytic acid. Soaking them overnight in salt water and boiling them for up to 3 hours the next day drastically reduces the concentration of phytic acid. The steady application of heat causes the phytic acid to degrade and break down, lessening its harmful effects on the body. Second, and this one is particularly good for grains, is fermentation. Take sourdough bread. At the time of writing this book, the whole world is in love with making its own sourdough bread. By fermenting a small amount of bread and water for a week, you allow natural yeast and bacteria to grow. This is what causes sourdough bread to rise. Additionally, pre-fermented foods such as yogurt and cheese are great additions to any meal and help combat antinutrients during digestion. In particular, the fermentation method is useful for combating phytic acid and lectins. Remember, most antinutrients are contained in the peel or the external layer of plants.

Conclusion

Antinutrients exist. What started as a diet craze eventually garnered scientific interest and antinutrients are finally being investigated for their harmful, and potentially beneficial, side effects on the human body. A primary concern of antinutrients is that they inhibit the uptake and absorption of essential vitamins and minerals from a balanced diet. Common antinutrients are phytic acid (phytate), oxalate, tannins, protease inhibitors, and lectins. In low quantities, these might not be harmful, but a high concentration of them can lead to severe side effects such as gut damage and malnutrition. Methods to reduce antinutrients in your diet will be explored further but two options to explore are boiling and fermentation. In the next chapter, we are going to look at the effects of plant foods on muscle growth and their relationship to muscle building.

CHAPTER 5: CAN YOU BUILD MUSCLE ON A VEGAN DIET?

There are a number of things that affect how muscle builds. Your body has some pretty amazing mechanisms in place to keep itself running. As we saw in an earlier chapter, your body can synthesize Vitamin D from UV rays when it's getting low. Although not in quite the same way, your body also has some amazing mechanisms in place to help you burn fat and build muscle, and there are things you can do to help these mechanisms along. Exercise, for example. A well-balanced regime focused on training muscle groups with a mix of isolation and compound exercises tones and strengthens muscle fibers. After working out and on rest days, you can supplement the work you put into your regime through your diet. Eating a balanced diet that is full of amino acids, protein, vitamins, and minerals gives your body the energy and building blocks it needs to heal and build itself up.

When lifting weights or performing bodyweight exercises, the way you perform the action can affect the way your muscles repair themselves. As a result of this form of exercise, your muscles start to grow and reshape themselves as a result of muscle hypertrophy. "Muscle hypertrophy" is the term for the increase and growth of muscle cells. It typically occurs when muscle fibers sustain damage or injury. While this might sound counterproductive, it's actually a well known mechanism. When building muscle through lifting weight, both mechanical damage and metabolic fatigue are necessary. The contractile proteins in your muscles need to generate force in order to counteract the resistance you're lifting. Structural damage to the muscles is simply a byproduct of this. In order to repair itself, the body fuses damaged fibers, which results in the increase of the mass and size of the muscle. The body releases hormones—such as testosterone, human growth hormone, and insulin growth factor—to assist with muscle repair. These hormones also stimulate growth.

When I refer to fatigue, I am talking about the body using up its supply of active transfer protein (ATP), the substance or energy that keeps your muscles contracted. ATP is also known as being the actual or raw energy source your body uses to do everything. This is why you might struggle to lift weights after a certain number of reps or when the weight gets too heavy. It is possible to train your body to use ATP more effectively, although this does depend on the fuel you provide your body with. The body takes what it needs from the food we give it. As we have covered, eating a plant-based diet can be severely lacking in nutrition. For this reason, a vegan diet needs to be heavily supplemented in order to receive proper nutrition. Dietary leucine and multivitamins, preferably non-synthetic versions are among the better options, although working with a registered dietician can help achieve some amazing results.

The most popular option and most effective one we are going to explore is protein powder. These are taken after a workout, usually mixed with water, milk, or a milk substitute. Bodybuilders take them together with BCAA supplements and post-workout mixes, while the average gym goer might drink a protein shake as a meal replacement. As the meat-free market has expanded, the protein industry has developed a variety of plant-based protein powders. However, there are some significant differences between animal-based protein powders and plant-based proteins, such as whey and hemp, respectively. Whey protein is the most well-known type of protein powder available on the market; it comes from dairy. Whey protein isolate has an average of 70g of protein per 100g, while just 30g of hemp protein can carry up to 15g of protein. These two proteins offer different health benefits and carry different nutritional values. As discussed in the previous chapter, antinutrients are also considered a protein and are counted in nutritional facts of foods, even though they are not absorbed. Later in the chapter, we will go through the different kinds of animal-based and plant-based proteins.

Can You Build Muscle On A Vegan Diet?

The question should be: can I build muscle if I'm avoiding the best foods to build muscle? So, with all of this in mind, I hope that the answer to this question is clear to you. This may surprise you, but it is possible to build muscle while on a vegan diet but only in certain conditions. As they say, "you must read and accept the terms and conditions". If you want to naturally build muscle on a plant-based diet, it is imperative to consume a lot of protein powders. It is basically impossible to build muscle by only consuming naturally occurring plant foods. This is because protein in most plants is not very bioavailable to the human body. Antinutrients, such as lectins, are not good proteins to build muscle yet it still counts as a protein on nutritional facts. Top athletes and body builders basically have to supplement steroids and/or testosterone with BCAAs to just maintain their physique on a plant-based diet. I also want to point out that self-advertised plant-based bodybuilders built most or all of their muscles when they were not plant-based.

I personally follow a meat-based keto plan because a plant-based diet doesn't work for me. However, I recognize that my diet might not be suitable for some people. For this reason, I want to explore a few options to assist people who enjoy a plant-based diet with building muscle and maintaining their health.

We're going to look at a few plant-based sources of protein and compare them with meat-based proteins. Something that people who enjoy a mixed diet have in common with plant-based diets is that both groups enjoy protein shakes to supplement their workouts. Protein shakes do offer an extra boost of protein that can assist with recovery but there are disadvantages to them, which we will get to later. The digestive tract makes use of enzymes and amino acids in the breakdown, or biosynthesis, of the nutrients we take in through food. One of these amino acids is called leucine.

Leucine is an amino acid used in the biosynthesis of proteins and has the capacity to directly stimulate myofibrillar muscle protein synthesis. That is to say, this amino acid helps you build muscle. It does this through activating rapamycin, which signals and aids in the regulation of the metabolism. Due to its part in protein synthesis, leucine can be taken as a supplement to treat muscle lesions, as a treatment for obesity and diabetes mellitus, or to assist with protein and energy deprivation. When prescribed, leucine has to be taken with a regulated food intake for it to be fully effective. The reason for this is that the underlying mechanisms are yet to be properly understood. For now, we know that it assists with muscle growth.

Protein

What Is Protein?

"Protein" is the catch-all term for macromolecules or long chains of amino acid residues. They are incredibly complex and play critical roles in the body. Proteins do a lot of the heavy lifting when it comes to the work in cells and structure, for example, and they play a huge role in the regulation of tissues and organs. Proteins are also an essential part of a proper diet.

One way a protein can be formed is when amino acids attach to one another to form long chains. In total, there are 20 types of amino acids and they can all link together in a variety of combinations to form different. It's this sequence that determines the structure of the protein and its specific function. A part of this is due to the DNA building blocks, also known as nucleotides, which give the amino acid its genetic sequence. On a chemical level, amino acids are made up of the carbon, hydrogen, oxygen, nitrogen, and sulfur. These organic compounds can combine in a variety of ways to form structures unique to specific amino acids.

Proteins play several key roles in the human body. One of the more important functions protein play is their role in the immune system. Immunoglobulin is a protein that binds to foreign bodies, such as bacteria and viruses, in order to protect the body. Messenger proteins also play a role in the transmission of chemical signals between cells, aiding in the transport of hormones to stimulate and coordinate biological processes between cells. Human growth hormone is a messenger protein because it plays a role in muscle development and growth. Structural component proteins, such as actin, play key roles in structure. On a smaller scale, actin assists with cellular structure but, on a larger scale, these proteins help the body move.

When we talk about "protein" in the sense of food, we mean the macronutrient. Macronutrients are nutrients that provide the greatest amount of calories or energy to a living organism. Broadly speaking, there are three classes: fat, carbohydrates, and protein. The body needs carbohydrates, such as sugar, to produce glucagon in order to keep the cells powered. The body needs fat because it's an essential source of fatty acids that the body cannot produce on its own and the body needs protein to build and maintain muscle mass in addition to vital functions, such as healing and cellular repair. Though I did mention that the body need carbohydrates for proper cell function, the body is technically able to produce glucose from amino acids (gluconeogenesis), which places carbohydrates at the non-essential nutrient category.

Protein, as a macronutrient, is so important to the diet because it contains a significant amount of amino acids that the body cannot produce on its own. Although there are 20 types of amino acids, there are 9 that are considered essential to the human diet. These are:

- Histidine
- Isoleucine
- Leucine
- Lysine
- Methionine
- Phenylalanine
- Threonine
- Tryptophan
- Valine

Most or all of these amino acids can be found in a variety of proteins, both animal- and plant-based. One animal-based protein that contains all 9 essential amino acids is albumen, commonly known as egg white. This is a cheap and readily available source of protein which, on average, contains about 3.6g of protein per egg white. The protein in egg whites is easy for the body to break down, assuming that egg white is not an allergen. At the start of the digestive tract is the mouth, where salivary amylase is produced. This, in addition to mastication, (chewing) breaks down and softens some of the proteins. As the protein is swallowed and enters the stomach, hydrochloric acid further denatures the proteins for absorption. As the amino acids are absorbed, they help fuel muscle mass and keep the immune system functioning and healthy.

There are multiple sources of protein. Eggs contain a lot of dietary fat in addition to amino acids and red meat such as a 12oz rump steak can contain up to 90g of protein. Red meat is also a great source of heme iron, as we covered earlier. In terms of plant-based protein, there are some pretty great sources if you know where to look. Chickpeas, for example, are so high in protein that the water from canned chickpeas can be used as a substitute for egg whites in most dishes. Keep in mind that chickpeas are a legume and will contain antinutrients, especially in the water of canned chickpeas. Properly preparing them is key if you want maximum bioavailability of the protein. Per 100g of chickpeas, you can expect to get 19g of protein, including antinutrients. You can even get isolated protein in protein powders. This most commonly occurs in whey protein, although it is rapidly becoming the norm in the plant-based protein sector. Getting processed plant protein powders is the best way to get more bioavailable protein as a plant-based dieter.

I want to take the next page or so to explore the benefits and downfalls of animal- and plant-based protein. We're going to cover some more sources of these proteins in addition to how the body responds to them.

Animal-Based Protein

Animal-based proteins are similar to the proteins we would find in the human body. Nutritionally, they are considered a source of complete protein because they contain all the amino acids that are necessary for the body to function properly. When we think of animal-based protein, we think of things like egg whites, red meat, poultry, and dairy products. Part of the cheesemaking process is to separate the two proteins, casein and whey. Whey is the liquid protein that remains once the cheese curds have been fully strained. This is what makes up about 20% of the milk before it goes to processing. It's also easily digestible while casein has a more complex structure and is harder for the body to break down.

The whey can be separated into three forms: whey isolate, whey concentrate, and whey hydrolysate. Most commonly used in protein powders, whey isolate and whey concentrate have different benefits and downsides. Downsides for both include nausea, stomach cramps, diarrhea, and headaches, although these symptoms typically occur if a large amount of whey is ingested in a short period of time. Whey concentrate contains about 70-80% protein and contains a little lactose (the sugar found in milk) in addition to some fat. On the other hand, whey isolate contains 90% protein or more and has less lactose. Whey concentrate contains most of the nutritional building blocks that naturally occur in whey before it's processed and is the option for people trying to lose weight or cut back on sugar. If you would like to focus on bulking up your muscles, whey isolate is the best option since it's practically all protein. However, whey isolate is not as nutritionally dense as whey concentrate.

A third type of animal-based protein might give you pause

for thought. As the world becomes more populated and nutrition becomes an increasing concern, environmental bodies have been researching the food of the future. One such innovation in nutrition is insect protein. Crickets are the most popular insect being used. Several brands have taken to mixing cricket protein with pea protein or serving it straight, describing the taste as "nutty" and "sweet." Additionally, it's high in several of the 9 essential amino acids, as well as being low in calories and high in Vitamin B12. Proponents of insect protein point to it being a much greener source of protein than modern factory farming as well as being much more sustainable. However, there are a few health concerns that are still being investigated given that insect protein is still relatively new. For example, the concern of allergens has risen as insects have been shown to trigger reactions in people with seafood allergies. Another concern related to what we covered in the previous chapter: it is still under investigation as to whether or not insect protein contains antinutrients. Some insects have been shown to contain trace amounts of phylate and other antinutrients, although many have dismissed this as negligible. Most insect protein powders are currently being used for animal feeds.

While protein powder makes a good supplement, the body cannot rely on it alone for everything it needs. Digestion helps the body maintain its metabolism and this is why eating food is so essential to maintaining a healthy, balanced diet especially when it comes to protein. You will find a lot of "all-in-one" or "all you need" branded meal replacement or protein shakes and, while these are great in a pinch, you could end up starving your body of everything it needs to function properly. Sources of animal protein, as previously mentioned, are considered nutritionally complete because the amino acids present in meat are so similar to the amino acids present in the human body.

Plant-Based Protein

Vegan protein powder became particularly popular around the year 2018. Although vegan alternatives have been growing steadily in availability since the late 1990s, 2018 saw a "breakthrough" for plant-based diets. Up until then, soy isolate and soy concentrate were the two main sources of protein in protein powders. The market has since expanded to include a wide variety of protein powder options including: pea protein, hemp protein, brown rice protein, and even mycoprotein. As with the whey protein market, these can be found in a variety of flavors and from various retailers. Plant-based proteins are referred to as "incomplete" proteins because they are either lower in or do not contain the 9 amino acids. However, this does not mean that the body cannot use them. It's simply the case that plant-based protein might be less bioavailable than animal-based protein.

Pea protein is made by drying out yellow split peas and then grinding them into a fine powder. After clearing away the starch and fiber, you're left with pea protein isolate. Proponents of pea protein often remark that it has a nicer taste than whey protein and while it contains fewer amino acids, it contains slightly more iron (non-heme iron). Approximately 20g of pea protein contains an average of 15g of protein and 5mg of non-heme iron while the same amount of whey protein contains 19g of protein and around 2mg of heme iron. Pea protein powder is ranked the highest in amino acid absorption for plant-based protein powders. Unfortunately, it is not a complete protein lacking in 2 amino acids. Adding a couple of eggs or a scoop of brown rice to your diet will undoubtably help to achieve a better amino acid profile in your diet. Most special diets, including gluten free and dairy free diets, can benefit from pea protein because it does not contain any of the top food allergens, including dairy, shellfish, cows' milk and soy. That being said, it should be avoided if you have an allergy or sensitivity towards peas. One downside to pea protein is that products made with it tend to be quite high in sodium with an average of 110-390mg per serving, depending on the product.

Another plant-based protein that is commonly used is a brown rice protein, which we will simply refer to as "rice protein." 25g of rice protein contains 24g of protein. Rice protein does contain amino acids but not all 9. Since rice protein is derived from brown rice, it is quite high in methionine. Again, with brown rice, the bran is kept in the mix. Where there's the outer protective layer of plant foods, antinutrients will follow. Brown rice is known to have arsenic residue left in it. If you are going to consume brown rice protein powder, make sure it is from the highest quality.

One last plant-based protein I want to explore is hemp protein. Before we continue, no hemp protein does not get you high, though it might be a good business idea. Hemp is made from Sativa, which is a cannabis plant bred specifically for industrial use, such as cloth, paper, and food.

While it does contain cannabidiol (CBD) and tetrahydrocannabinol (THC), the amounts are so negligible that they may as well not be counted. Every part of this plant is used, including the seeds from which hemp protein is derived. To turn the seeds into protein, the oil is extracted from the seeds, which are then ground into a fine powder. It has a nutty, earthy taste. The essential amino acid profile of hemp protein is equivalent to egg whites and, when compared to other plant proteins, is much easier to digest. This makes it a good supplement for anyone suffering from stomach issues or conditions such as IBS. A few side effects have been reported, including headaches and stomach aches.

The last few years (2017-2021) have also seen a rise in vegan bodybuilders such as Jehina Malik and Karl Bruder. I do believe that these guys built most of their muscle before ever going vegan and who knows what else they have been doing to increase muscle growth. Point is, it's a far stretch to say that a vegan diet made them build all this muscle. Being vegan and a bodybuilder might seem like opposite ends of a spectrum but the answer to building muscle as a vegan is to load up on plant protein powders and take supplements as necessary. Notice how, as a vegan or plant-based dieter, you need to consume processed plant foods to build muscle. Some people might not like what I'm about to say but, I believe it is impossible to gain major muscles with purely unprocessed natural vegan foods.

Processed protein powders have the added benefit of having an increased protein bioavailability profile while also having less antinutrients. Relying on unprocessed natural plant foods for muscle growth will not get you far. Not only does fiber in your diet reduces protein absorption, but it also reduces the time protein stays in your gut. Some plant foods also contain protein that are just purely undigestible for the human body.

Unavailable Protein - Gluten

Although the body can process some plant-based proteins, it cannot absorb all of them. This next protein I'm about to discuss is one of the most common food intolerances. Gluten is a general term for protein storage in grains. More specifically, it is found in barley, wheat, and rye. If you have celiac disease, this is the substance that triggers the inflammatory immune response in the body. These toxic proteins are rich in two amino acids: proline and glutamine. As a group, they are known as prolamins. Each grain has its own specific prolamin fraction: wheat has gliadin, rye has secalin, and barley has hordein.

Prolamins are abundant in proline and glutamine, both of which the body struggles to digest. The normal digestion process breaks up the long strands of amino acids into smaller peptide strands, which can be broken down further and absorbed through the intestine to be transported throughout the body. The body is incapable of breaking down the long strands of amino acids found in gluten. This is due to three specific gluten peptides that trigger the T-cell response, which leads to inflammation. Due to the high proline and glutamine content, toxic oligopeptides form. These are proteins with up to ten amino acids and are present in the small intestine. Since they cannot be broken down by the enzymes in the body, they simply stay in the small intestine and cause the erosion of the intestinal lining.

This is what happens in people who suffer from celiac disease. If you do not suffer from celiac disease, you will most likely be just fine. The body simply cannot use the proteins stored in gluten because it's impossible to digest. While your body might want the carbohydrates in the toast you have for breakfast or that pasta you are enjoying for dinner, the gluten it contains is completely unavailable to you.

Supplementation

Now that we have gone through protein powders, I feel that we should get back to the vegan diet. Adding a scoop or two of protein powder to your diet will help you out a lot but the overall diet is so lacking that it's harder to build muscle while eating a plant-based diet. Animal-based proteins are easier to digest and have a stronger anabolic effect than plant-based proteins. Anabolic effects are produced by anabolic hormones, the main type being hormonal in nature. Several key hormones come into play when building muscle: human growth hormone, brain-derived neurotrophic factor, insulin, testosterone, and insulin-like growth factor.

Human growth hormone assists with muscle repair and growth; brain-derived neurotrophic factor shifts the proportion of muscle fibers; insulin assists in the production of glucagon, which powers cells; insulin-like growth factor stimulates growth and decreases blood glucose levels;

testosterone increases neurotransmitters and encourages tissue growth. All of these hormones are produced by the human body and can be supplemented if required. The metabolism is the sum of all processes that occur in the human body and it can be affected by hormone levels.

In general, protein powders are processed in such a way to make them more absorbable. They're a great supplement but are not meant to replace entire meals. The best thing you can do for your body and your hormones is to eat a balanced diet. I don't think I can stress that enough. One of the things your body needs to be able to digest food and properly break down proteins, in addition to leucine, are B vitamins. Vitamin B6, known by its chemical name as pyridoxal 5 phosphate, is crucial for protein metabolism and is mostly found in meats. This is key to the biosynthesis of amino acids because it acts as a coenzyme in all transamination reactions. Transamination reactions are chemical reactions that occur when an amino group is transferred to a keto acid in order to form new amino acids. Part of the process is the deamination of amino acids. In biochemistry, the enzymes responsible for this are transaminases or aminotransferases.

As you might be able to glean from the context, these processes are incredibly important for our overall health. However, they cannot happen if there are no protein strands to break down. As I keep saying, protein powders are not meant to replace a meal. While it is true that they can provide a source of protein to supplement your daily intake, the protein in them is simply not adequate for the human body. Naturally occurring proteins that occur in animal products such as eggs, red meat, poultry, and seafood are much easier for the body to break down because of pepsin. Pepsin is an enzyme released in the stomach. Its primary purpose is to break down the peptide strands in protein and it works best with animal proteins. Pepsin is acidic in nature. Due to this, the stomach coats itself with a mucus-like membrane to prevent itself from being digested along with the food. Some people might not be able to produce enough pepsin, as is common in plant-based diets, so pepsin supplements are available either over the counter or by prescription to aid with digestion.

Another form of supplementation is through a good, old-fashioned multivitamin. There are many brands available, some catered to men and some catered to women. Multivitamins get a bad reputation because, in theory, you should be able to get everything you need from a balanced diet. However, as we have seen, this is not always possible, particularly if you eat only plant-based food. A multivitamin, as the name suggests, contains all of the minerals and vitamins the human body requires. They are not meant to replace a full meal, they are meant to give your body an extra source in case it doesn't get everything it needs from food. If your diet is already varied and balanced, chances are you don't need it. For this reason, you should seek the advice of a nutritionist or dietitian before taking one. Try aiming for B vitamins that are advertised as "complex" and try avoiding synthetic versions of vitamins.

Before we continue into the next chapter, I want us to revisit leucine. For a quick recap: leucine is one of the 9 essential amino acids, it helps with protein synthesis and the synthesis of active transport protein, and it plays a role in the metabolism. Leucine also has another function. It's one of the three block-chain amino acids, commercially known as BCAAs. The body cannot produce block-chain amino acids (henceforth, BCAAs) on its own, it needs to take them in through ingestion. If you've heard of BCAAs or seen them on the shelf at a grocery store or fitness outlet, you would probably assume they were something that body-builders and weightlifters take ritualistically to achieve impossibly large biceps. You'd, almost, be right. Supplemental BCAAs are taken as a part of a weightlifting or bodybuilding regime because their "main" effect is muscle gain. You can find protein powders that have added BCAAs. These have the worst side effects, regardless of whether they're animal- or plant-based. You can experience headaches, diarrhea, migraines, heart palpitations, and a whole host of other side effects if your body isn't used to them. You can get leucine as a supplement on its own, so the effects won't be quite as intense. A little stomach pain is normal and you might notice that your muscles start to get a little tougher as you workout. Studies have shown that supplemental leucine can actually increase lean muscle mass and speed up the metabolism to burn fat more effectively. Of course, it's unknown if leucine directly causes this latter effect or if it's a result of exercise.

Conclusion

Protein powders should be treated as supplements only and are not reliable sources of nutrition. However, on a plant-based diet, protein powders are a must as the natural unprocessed plant foods have a very low bioavailability rate. In order to get the most out of a plant-based diet, heavy supplementation is required due to the severe lack of nutrients present in plant foods. There are a large variety of animal- and plant-based protein powders; the main animal-based powders available are whey protein, egg protein powder and insect protein, while the market for plant-based protein powders has expanded to include hemp, rice, and pea protein as alternatives to traditional soy protein. These powders, regardless of origin, have been processed in such a way as to make them easier to digest. For this reason, they are supplemental only. The body needs natural sources of nutrition to function properly. Supplementation is useful in achieving an end goal but should not be the main form of nutrition. Taking multivitamins can aid in replenishing nutrients lost or used through exercise and supplemental leucine can assist with muscle growth. Taking BCAAs in the form of fortified protein powders can have dangerous side effects, so consulting a medical or dietary professional is the best course of action.

In the next chapter, we are going to look at the short-term and long-term effects of going on a plant-based diet. This is probably going to be the longest chapter in the book, so get comfortable.

CHAPTER 6: SYMPTOMS TO EXPECT

Converting to a plant-based diet does have its positive effects in the beginning. You do feel a little more energized, your carbon footprint goes down by a margin, and you get to explore a wide variety of new cuisines. Vegetarian and vegan cooking is a challenge that a lot of people take up. The influx of plant foods is enough to overwhelm your body and mind, making you feel healthier when you are actually starving your body. Going to the gym will feel better at first but, over the course of a few short months, you will begin to notice some shocking changes. Without proper protein intake, you will lose muscle mass. At first, you might think you're losing weight, but, by the time you notice that you're losing muscle, it's going to be an uphill climb to gain it back.

A lot of people go plant-based in order to lose weight. This, actually, is something that going plant-based can help with but not for the reasons they think. In addition to losing muscle mass, another way that a plant-based diet "helps" you lose weight is through malnutrition. Malnutrition is an umbrella term for deficiencies, excesses, or imbalances in a diet. Plant-based diets, specifically veganism, are lacking in so many vitamins and minerals that you might as well be just shoot yourself in the foot as well.

Sugar is present in just about everything. Generally speaking, if it ends in the suffix "-ose," it's a sugar. Plants are so full of naturally occurring sugars that your body doesn't know what to do with them. For the first few weeks, your body produces a little more insulin to keep up with the sudden influx of sugar but, the longer this goes on, the higher the chances of developing metabolic syndrome, also known as insulin resistance. As we will see later, the excess of fiber might help get your bowels moving in the short-term but the long term will be much less appealing.

These are just a couple of the symptoms to expect when you switch to a plant-based diet. At the root of these issues, and the ones to come, is poor nutrition. In the chapter that follows, we're going to look at how to overcome these issues. For now, let's get into what you can expect when you go plant-based.

Early Symptoms

Transitioning from a standard American diet to veganism or plant-based diet will definitely give you a boost in the short term. This happens because of the increase of Vitamin C, antioxidants and possibly because of the removal of vegetable oils. A standard American diet consists of a lot of processed foods which, in bulk, is bad for the digestive system, heart, and brain. Going plant-based for a short time is actually a good way to reverse this and give your body a chance to recover from your normal standard American diet. The first symptoms you might experience are bloating and flatulence. Then, fatigue will eventually sneak itself in your day-to-day life. Unfortunately, when carried on for too long, things will really start to head south.

Bloating and Flatulence

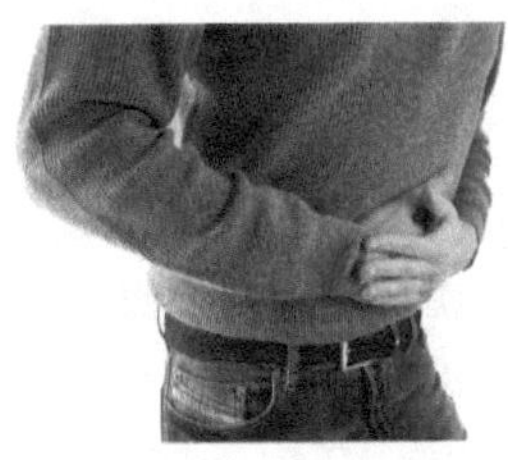

Due to the sudden influx of fiber, you're going to experience certain gastronomical abnormalities, which might seem beneficial at first, but will quickly become intolerable. Your bowel movements will be much more frequent. While this gets rid of the excess waste, it can also prevent your body from absorbing what little nutrition you have taken in through your food. The staples of a plant-based diet include beans and lentils, both ostensibly high in protein. These two common canned goods form the bulk of most vegan meat replacements and can take center stage in a significant number of vegetarian and vegan dishes.

We all know the rhyme: "Beans beans, they're good for your heart; the more you eat, the more you fart." The latter half of this rhyme is much truer than you think. Beans are high in sugar and one of these sugars is called raffinose. It's a complex sugar that the body doesn't like to digest because it's difficult to break down. The bacteria in your large and lower intestines love breaking down sugar. Raffinose passed through your intestines and is broken down into hydrogen, carbon dioxide, and methane gas by the bacteria there. The more beans you eat as part of a plant-based diet, the more raffinose your body will struggle to break down and the more bloated and flatulent you will become.

Raffinose aside, a vegan diet is high in leafy green vegetables. Vegetables contain a lot of fiber that can be good for your overall gut health. Fiber, commonly known as "roughage," helps us feel fuller for longer. In part, this is why vegans tend to feel less hungry in the beginning, but we'll cover that soon enough. Having a huge serving of collard greens with every meal is hard on the body. This results in bloating. Bloating can occur for two main reasons: trapped gas from, fermented fibers, making you feel "stuffed," or you are experiencing disturbances in your digestive system. The second of these two causes is usually due to food intolerance but it can be attributed to a plant-based diet as well. Unlike water retention, bloating involves a large amount of solids, liquids, and gas present in your digestive system.

The only thing that can make you stop bloating is to reduce fiber intake or just completely avoid it for a while. Common practice for vegans is to have a large glass of water alongside a meal heavy on the greens to prevent bloating in addition to cutting down on their serving of greens. Something a lot of new vegans do at the start of their new regime is to overload on the vegan meat replacements and vegetables. This is not the way to go. If you aren't a physically active person, eating a large amount of food in one sitting is a recipe for bloating and discomfort. To prevent this from happening, simply eat less fiber rich foods. A new diet, regardless of whether it's plant-base or animal-based, is a prime opportunity to practice meal prepping and portion control.

Acid Reflux/GERD

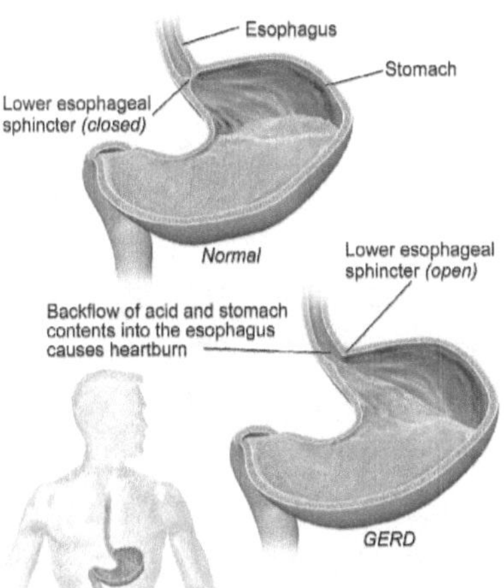

Gastroesophageal Reflux Disease (GERD)

In the past, it has long been taught that acid reflux was due to high stomach acid. As a treatment, people would take anti-acid pills to combat this annoying condition. But in reality, this condition seems to be caused by low stomach acid instead of high stomach acid. This valve seems to only close properly once it senses a high acidity PH. GERD happens when the lower esophageal sphincter does not, or is unable to, close properly. This allows stomach acid and bile to rise up into the low esophagus and cause heartburn. GERD is also caused by frequent acid reflux and some common symptoms are as follows: chest pain, difficulty swallowing, sensation of a lump in your throat, burning sensation in your chest when lying down, and chronic cough. A plant-based diet, processed meat replacements aside, seems to help because it can act as an anti-acid. A diet high in fiber will lower stomach acid due to the increased surface area. But the true reason this problem occurs is because of low stomach acid, which plant-based dieters struggle with because of their bulky meals and the fact that fiber has such a big surface area.

A plant-based diet is by default less calorie-dense. The human body requires 1800-2500 calories on average and, depending on one's sex, in order to maintain functionality. People who track their calories aim for a calorie deficit in order to lose weight or a calorie surplus if they want to gain muscle. When your diet consists of plants, which contain barely anything of nutritional value, you are likely to get much hungrier than normal. Something that occurs as a result is eating in excessive amounts, which requires your stomach to produce more acid. Your lower esophageal sphincter might open up to relieve the pressure on your stomach, which results in acid reflux.

Heartburn is a problem regardless of diet, it just so happens that vegans are not immune to it and can potentially become a problem. A bland plant-based diet can help alleviate the symptoms but it is not the cure. I would like to offer a few general tips to anyone who might struggle with heartburn. First, cut back on caffeine, particularly coffee and black tea. The tannins in tea are not good for the stomach. Second, lower your fiber intake as it will reduce your stomach acidity. Third, try not to drink water while eating and wait at least an hour before drinking after your meal. The trick is to drink a lot of water before your meal. This helps because you will not feel thirsty while eating and you will not dilute you stomach acid. Forth, have a sip on some apple cider vinegar. This will help acidify your stomach to a good PH. Finally, sit upright or otherwise elevate your upper body and breathe from the stomach. This will relieve the pressure on your stomach and shift it into a different position.

Ultimately, you should seek medical advice if acid reflux or heartburn persists, it can cause a myriad of health problems later in life. If left untreated, acid reflux can cause stomach ulcers to develop and, in extreme cases, irreparable damage to the esophagus and stomach lining. For this reason, if symptoms persist, see your doctor immediately.

Excessive Hunger and Cravings

Just like pregnant women, vegans will often experience excessive hunger and pain. The reason this happen for pregnant women are quite different and self-explanatory compared to vegans. Because plant-based diets are so lacking in nutrition, the body will start to crave for more food. Since diet is mostly comprised of sugar as the energy source, it is almost part of every single meal. Blood glucose being constantly on a rollercoaster ride going up and down happens very often for vegans. After a sugary meal of fruits or starches, hyperglycemia occurs for the first hour and then hypoglycemia creeps in to make you hungry again. Cravings can also occur due to malnutrition.

As we covered much earlier in this book, changing to a plant-based diet leads to deficiencies in several essential vitamins and minerals. Taking mineral supplements will most likely get rid of a deficiency, but for things like B12 and omega 3 fatty acids, it can be much more difficult. The body will start to crave the sources of nutrition that it's missing. Red meat, for example, is a common craving in people who struggle with iron deficiency anemia. Cravings can also include salmon or trout to counteract the need for omega 3 fatty acids. In order to circumvent this, you have to keep on top of your protein intake. By doing this, you will give your body a better source of energy and something to work on digesting for a longer time than just plant foods.

Hormonal Problems

People who eat a plant-based diet go into it without properly understanding the nutrition required to maintain healthy hormonal balances. Hormonal cycles, most notably the menstrual cycle and testosterone cycle, are affected by nutrition. The food we eat, both in quantity and quality, can significantly affect the production and secretion of hormones in the body. Estrogen levels, for example, can be affected by soy protein. Testosterone levels can be affected by chia seeds. When people make a drastic switch to a plant-based diet, they often do so with limited research into what they're getting into. They hear the usual buzzwords like "healthy" and "eco-friendly" but they don't stop to think how it could affect their body and as a result they don't look into the necessary supplementation they will inevitably require.

There have been several studies into how a vegan diet affects male hormones. Some studies claim that a plant-based diet with proper supplementation can enhance or maintain healthy testosterone levels, while other studies show disturbances in the testosterone cycle. One study, from which the term "soy boy" is derived, showed that a group of men who drank soy isolate protein experienced a drop in testosterone after 54 days. The group only consisted of 35 men and, of course, did not represent the larger male population. Human research is still ongoing in this area, but I think we should also consider the elevated amount of pesticides and chemicals that can act as an estrogen. Glyphosate is a popular pesticide used on all sorts of crops and is very well known to have estrogenic effects on humans once consumed. One study suggest that glyphosate is around half as 17 b-estradiol, the most potent estrogen. A lack of cholesterol is the diet will also lead to a decrease in steroid hormones, which includes testosterone and estrogen.

One strange benefit of a plant-based diet is an easier transition into menopause. It is currently speculated that lower levels of estrogen are a reason for this. That being said, women who are not yet menopausal can still experience an irregular menstrual cycle. A lack of iron in the diet is responsible for this and it can actually amplify premenstrual syndrome. In particular, cramping and irritability can become much more intense. Heavier menstruation, too, can also become an issue. As is becoming a common theme, malnutrition is as a result of a diet lacking in essential vitamins and minerals.

Inflammation

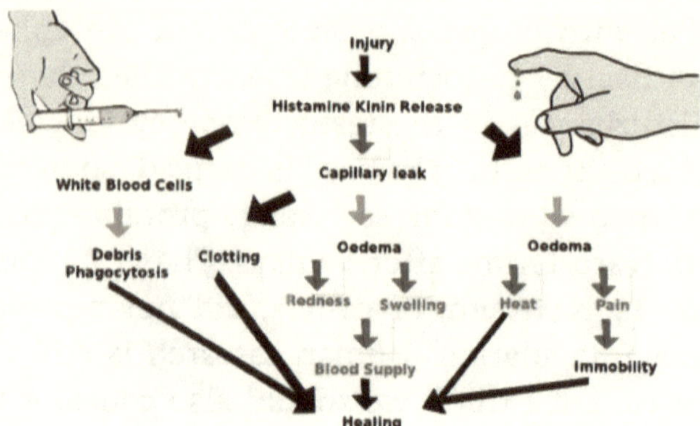

The inflammation process occurs when tissues are damaged and infected by bacteria, viruses, or other pathogens. Damaged cells release histamine, bradykinin, and prostaglandins and blood rushes to the injured area to speed up the healing process. At the beginning of a plant-based diet, and throughout, you risk removing vital nutrients, which make it more difficult for the body to heal. Healing is a taxing process for the body, which is why breaking an arm or recovering from a would makes you feel exhausted.

Inflammation is the body's natural response to injury and infection although it can be the root cause of other conditions. Possibly the best known inflammatory condition is arthritis, which is characterized by a swelling of the joints. Cardiovascular diseases, cancer, and chronic inflammatory disease are also linked to problems with inflammation and can be made worse with a plant-based diet.

The results regarding the effects of a plant-based diet on inflammatory conditions, like arthritis, are mixed. Some evidence suggests that levels of CRP (C-reactive protein), a protein associated with the inflammation processes in the body, might be reduced as a result of a plant-based diet. On the other hand, studies have also associated a plant-based diet with increased levels of the inflammatory biomarker IL-6. IL-6 is an important biomarker because it plays a role in fever and the acute phase response; it also helps in the formation of B cells. This could be due to lower levels of calcium, Vitamin B12, and Vitamin D. Eating a diet consisting of gut-wrenching compounds and inflammatory foods also add up to the inflammation.

Depression and Anxiety

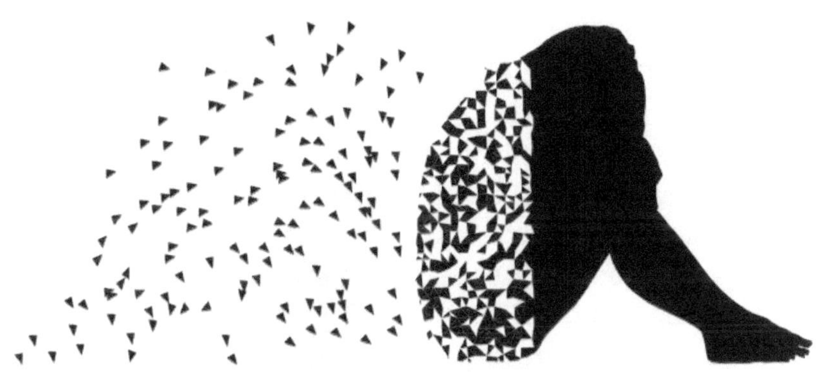

What we eat can have a significant effect on our mental health. According to a study, "gut microbiome diversity has a strong association with mood-relating behaviors". Now what the heck does that mean? Diversity used in this context refers to the diversity of bacteria and fungi in your gut. The link between depression and diet has been studied to such an extent that an entirely new field called "nutritional psychiatry" has developed around it.

A bad gut microbiome will create bad psychological side-effects, including depression and anxiety. It has also been shown time and time again that a fecal microbiota transplant will change the patient's psychological behavior. A FMT of a depressed individual to a healthy individual will cause the healthy patient to experience depression and vice-versa. Someone who's not suffering from depression nor anxiety can give a FMT to someone with those symptoms and will see an improvement over their depression. This sounds like some complete voodoo science but the data on this seems clear. The gut and the brain have such a strong link together that some people even consider the gut as the second brain.

With that being said, what is a good microbiome and what is not? The goal is to have the most divers ecosystem in your gut while keeping it in control. You want as many different strains of healthy bacteria as possible. Too many bacteria in your small intestine will create a problem known as SIBO, which is usually caused by a diet high in sugar and carbohydrates. Remember when we talked about antinutrients and the gut damaging effect they have? This is another culprit to depression and anxiety symptoms. Stress and going through difficult moments have also been shown to damage the gut microbiome.

Depression is characterized by lethargy, low mood, increased or decreased appetite and changes in sleeping pattern. Anxiety is characterized by extreme or intense worry about any number of events, real or imagined, and can have multiple physical symptoms including feeling restless, irritable or easily tired.

The physical symptoms of depression and anxiety can easily be attributed to nutritional deficiencies. Vitamin B12, which is a key nutrient which affects the metabolism.

One of the symptoms of B12 deficiency is irritability. Poor appetite and lethargy are both symptoms of Vitamin D deficiency. If you are experiencing any kind of mental health issues it is vital that you speak with a mental health professional or GI doctor in order to address underlying issues. You can also visit viome.com to get your microbiome tested, though I don't have any previous experience with this company so I can't talk much more about them.

Weight Gain

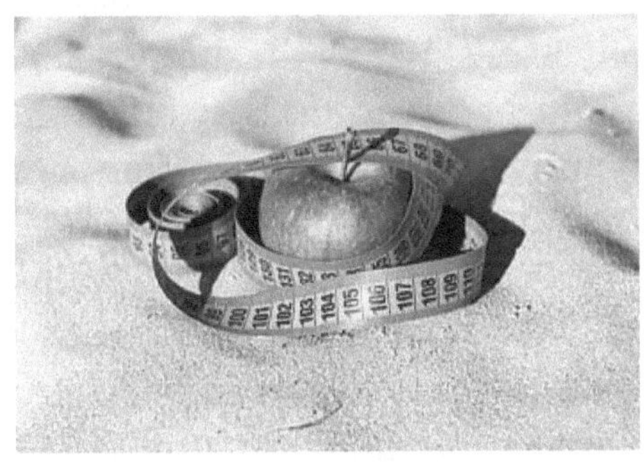

Many people go vegetarian or vegan because they think it will help them lose weight. While this will happen in the form of muscle loss, it is not the case with body fat. As discussed in the previous chapter, people who eat a predominantly plant-based diet will suffer muscle loss. This occurs on their overall body but also appears in the face as collagen loss and eye bags. Gaining weight is surprisingly easy on a plant-based diet. As we have already covered, you need a calorie surplus in order to gain weight and this is useful for those who want to gain muscle mass. However, a calorie surplus only works when you are doing heavy resistance training. There are several mistakes people make when they turn to a plant-based diet. Because plant foods are lacking in nutritional value, it is easier than you might think to eat too much. Refined carbohydrates, particularly in the form of pasta, are a staple of many plant-based and college diets. On a molecular level, refined wheat has become so simple and easy to digest that the body does not register that it has eaten anything at all in the hours after eating. Blood sugar goes down much sooner than if you had eaten a balanced meal. As a result, the body triggers the hunger mechanisms, causing cravings for calorie-dense foods, which just pack on the pounds.

Plants are mostly made up of carbohydrates. Carbohydrates can be an important macronutrient depending on how active you are. Tracking your macros through a fitness app can be a helpful way to lose weight but, what people do not realize about most plant-based diets, is just how easy it is to overindulge on carbohydrates. When the diet is overindulgent in carbohydrates, the body responds by bloating. Trapped gas, food solids, and even water retention can cause the abdomen to protrude outward like there's a basketball under your shirt. The reason why someone gains weight in the first place is because of a certain hormone called insulin. This hormone allows glucose to enter cells to then be used as energy. Another role this hormone serves is to store extra calories as belly or visceral fat. Since a "plant-based" diet tend to steer more towards sugar and carbohydrates, insulin becomes very present and therefore it becomes very easy to store fat. Estrogen is also another hormone that encourages fat gain. Phytoestrogen, meaning estrogen found in plants, are common in a vegan diet, soy being the best example. Overconsuming those plant foods high in phytoestrogen will promote fat gain. Our modern world is filled with estrogenic compounds (BPA) found in foods, plastic containers even a regular shopping receipt has BPA on it. If you think you are suffering from hormonal problems, it might be worth your time research this.

Another way in which a plant-based diet causes weight gain is through excessive plant-based junk food. It may not immediately seem obvious but a lot of plant-based meat replacements are highly processed and contain shockingly high levels of fat and carbohydrates. New vegans and vegetarians hear "plant-based" and assume "healthy" when this is not the case. A healthy diet is one where your relationship with food is healthy and sustainable, while the food you give your body is also nutritionally dense and varied. Just because a vegan "beef" burger is plant-based, that doesn't make it healthy. Look at the packaging on any meat replacement and you are sure to see high levels of salt, fat, sugar, and carbohydrates. All four of these things are substances that the body craves so it's easy to overindulge. The way to resolve this is to completely overhaul your eating habits. Notice when you reach for the junk food and ask yourself if there's a healthier version you could eat.

Depending on your definition of "plant-based," there are many different kinds of diets. Lacto-ovo vegetarians and flexitarians (which is often included under the "plant-based" umbrella) are probably the healthiest of them. Lacto-ovo vegetarians have access to all nine essential amino acids and sources of iron that are lacking in a vegan diet, while flexitarians are able to "pick and choose" when they want to eat meat. Going through the different categorizations of plant-based diets is a topic for another book but I wanted to include it because there are variances in the different diets. Part of why people gain weight on a plant-based diet is the lack of proper research. They just throw out all of their animal-based products and eat green leafy vegetables and fruit at every meal. Researching the different types of plant-based diets can save a lot of headaches, both figurative and literal, in the long-term, especially when it comes to maintaining a healthy weight. Understanding the different sources of protein and whey protein shakes might not be the best way to up your protein intake, can be a valuable tool in your nutritional backpack.

Lastly, I want to look at portion control. This is related to the above point about overindulgence and processed foods. Regardless of the diet you eat, you might be tempted by an extra scoop of ice cream or a brownie. This is no less true of a plant-based diet. Another assumption made about plant-based alternatives to common desserts is that they are lower in calories when this is simply not the case. Again, check the back of the packaging and you will see that the plant-based alternative contains just as many, if not more, calories than the non-vegan alternative. Indulging in sweets every now and then is fine and part of a healthy diet but do not assume that the words "plant-based" are a synonym for "healthy."

Hyperhomocysteinemia

The amino acid homocysteine is produced when proteins are broken down. When produced, Vitamins B12 and 6, along with folic acid, break it down to synthesize it into a protein the body can use. High levels of homocysteine typically means Vitamin B12 or folate deficiency. When homocysteine levels get too high, this can result in arterial damage and cardiovascular disease. Mineral and vitamin deficiencies share a variety of symptoms, including fatigue and dizziness. This is no less true of hyperhomocysteinemia. Folate deficiency is a little more subtle but the main symptom to look out for is growth problems in young children and mouth sores in adults.

Hyperhomocycteinemia has a variety of causes. While it's often attributed to Vitamin B12 and 6 deficiencies, it can also be caused by low levels of thyroid hormones, genetics, and kidney disease. Some medications, such as metformin and cholestyramine, can also interfere with mineral absorption, which results in high homocysteine levels. Metformin is a medication often prescribed to diabetics to help maintain high blood glucose. While diabetes has a strong genetic component, it can also be caused by significant dietary changes. Too many carbohydrates, as we have seen with a plant-based diet, often means too much blood sugar, which causes insulin to be produced at a high rate. If you need to take a medication like metformin, you need to keep on top of your homocysteine levels.

Hyperhomocycteinemia can lead to a wide variety of health complications. Heart disease and stroke are perhaps the two most serious. In addition to this, a variety of other complications are present: osteoporosis (thinning of the bones), atherosclerosis (build up of fatty deposits in the arterial wall), venous thrombosis (blood clots in the veins), thrombosis (clotting in the blood vessels), and to a more extreme extent, dementia and Alzheimer's. Vitamin B12 plays a crucial role in the creation of red blood cells, which keeps the body and mind healthy. Without this vital vitamin, the risk of contracting the listed health complications only increases. Since Vitamin B12 is only found in animal-based foods, it's borderline impossible to source it naturally in a plant-based diet, hence the need for supplementation. For this, you would have to really keep on top of your Vitamin B12 supplements and seek medical advice as necessary.

Skin Problems

Alot of skin problems are prevalent in a plant-based diet. Foods which have a high glycemic index such as refined carbohydrates have long been associated with skin issues. A food's glycemic index affects your blood sugar. In general, the higher the glycemic index the higher the glucose spike and the faster the crash. Plant-based diets rely on processed and refined carbohydrates to form the bulk of meat replacements. While plant-based diets have the potential to benefit your skin for the short-term, in the long term your skin could suffer a significant amount of damage. One common and serious condition that might occur is acne. Though I will write a book on acne eventually, I will give you guys a quick sneak peek right here. As an ex-acne sufferer myself, I successfully resolve it through diet and probiotic supplements. Acne can be caused by multiple factors, such as gut damage, allergens (dairy for example), B vitamin deficiency but also the constant blood sugar influx. The constant influx of refined carbohydrates and processed oils, when coupled with the Vitamin B12 deficiency, causes the body to amplify production of androgen, a hormone that is present in both males and females. This hormone regulates "male" characteristics such as body hair. High levels of androgen can also affect the skin, making it more or less oily, which can lead to subsequent breakouts of acne.

The common factor in all health conditions, even something as apparently superficial as one's complexion, is a deficiency in vitamins and minerals. Fruits and vegetables, in addition to other plant foods, have been bred to have significantly more sugar than what our bodies are capable of processing. What little nutritional value there is in something like an apple or an orange, for example, can be overlooked as the body fights against the influx of sugar it receives. People who are new to a plant-based diet often forget to source decent nutritional supplements. You may have noticed that supplementation has become a common solution to all of the problems I have listed and this is because it's really the only way to give the body what it needs. Most people plan their meals, but the meals themselves become routine, which means that your body gets used to certain levels of nutrition. This lack of variety leads the body to become complacent and store up excess sugars as fat in the adipose layer beneath the skin. This leads to another cause of skin problems: weight gain.

We have already covered weight gain as a side effect so I won't revisit it. When you gain weight, certain changes to the skin occur, most notable of which being that it loses moisture. This could be in the form of excessive sweating or it could be from being stretched out. When the skin gets dry, it becomes scaly and starts to crack. This can actually be treated through the use of omega 3 supplements or skin creams that are rich in Vitamin E. However, these can be a costly solution in the long term. One significant cause of dry skin is a lack of fatty acids in the diet. Omega 3 fatty acids aid in the production of sebum, which keeps the skin healthy and "water proof," meaning that it doesn't allow water to enter the body through the skin. This is why excessive washing with alcohol-heavy soaps can lead to dry and itchy skin. "Vegan-friendly" skin problems are often packed full of alcohol, which strips away the sebum and leaves the skin vulnerable to the elements.

Dental Problems

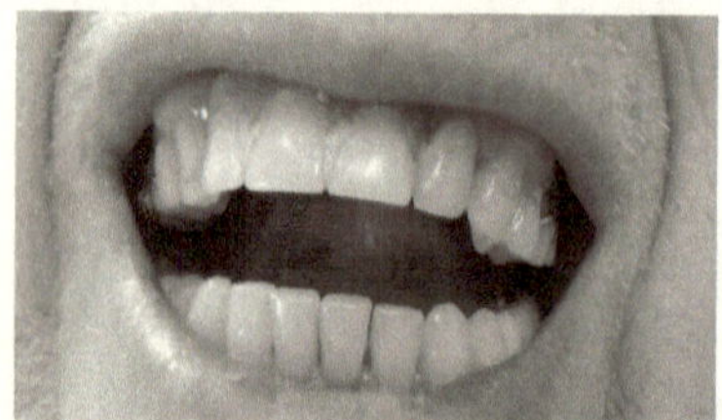

Studies have shown that a plant-based diet can lead to a higher risk of tooth decay. Tooth decay occurs when the buildup of plaque on the teeth converts sugar into acid. Currently, it is speculated that the reason for this is that plant-based diets contain more acidic and sugary foods. Plaque forms when the bacteria inside the mouth mixes with starch and sugars that are present in food. Since plant-based foods are full of starch and sugar, anyone who follows a plant-based diet has to take extra care of their teeth. When left untreated, plaque can lead to a lot of dental problems. Holes in the teeth, also known as cavities, occur as a result. Additionally, the risk of gum disease skyrockets as a direct result of plaque. Due to the lack of minerals, essential amino acids as well as Vitamin K2 in most plant-based diets, teeth are unable to remineralize. To put it simply, tooth remineralization is the dental healing process. When the enamel on your teeth erodes, the body draws calcium, phosphate, and on occasion fluoride ions to the tooth in order to strengthen and remineralize the enamel. A Vitamin D3 deficiency makes this process much more taxing on the body, leaving the teeth in such a state of disrepair that they begin to fall out.

The gums also suffer as a result of a plant-based diet. Arginine is an amino acid that plays a role in the breakdown of plaque in the mouth. It is most often found in meat, poultry, fish and dairy, although trace amounts are found in vegan sources like pumpkin seeds. Sugar is also, and always, a major concern when it comes to teeth. The bacteria that live in our mouths love it, it's their favorite food. Eating a lot of starchy, processed foods causes these bacteria to thrive and, as a result, they begin to eat away at the teeth and settle into microabrasions (small cuts) in the mouth as well as the gaps between the teeth, leading to diseased gums. Symptoms of gum disease include red, swollen gums and bleeding when brushing your teeth. Bad breath can also be a symptom because of the amount of bacteria that collects in the gum lining. Gum disease itself has a straightforward treatment: go to your dentists and get a professional cleaning, then brush and floss twice a day and rinse with mouthwash before you go to bed. In more severe cases, medical intervention might be required.

Recovery Time

I'm using "recovery time" as an umbrella term. This term can be used to reference any number of things, including the recovery time after a period of heavy exercise and the time spent recovering from injury or illness. People who enjoy a balanced diet with a variety of foods rich in all of the vitamins, minerals, and amino acids can expect to recover from the flu in around two to two and a half weeks, depending on the severity of the infection and treatment options available. Recovering from a cold can take as little as three days. When you break a bone, you might be given calcium supplements regardless of your diet in an attempt to speed up the recovery process.

Continuing with the example of a broken bone, let's say that a patient has a clean break on their humerus, the long bone which extends from the shoulder to the elbow. In addition to the bone, the soft tissue and surrounding muscles will likely become inflamed from the rush of blood to the area. Not only this, they might sustain superficial damage from the impact which caused the break. The body has a variety of healing processes and, for a broken bone, this requires the two broken edges to be placed together so that they can "knit" themselves back into one piece. Healing takes up a lot of energy from the body, which is why nutrients are so important when you're recovering from any sort of injury. A broken bone can take up to 8 weeks to heal fully. Depending on your general health, this can take longer than expected, as is the case in people who struggle with malnutrition and calcium deficiency. Since the bones require a lot of calcium and Vitamin D and K2 to remain healthy, you can imagine how much more it would take to get them to heal efficiently.

Recovering from an infection, like with the flu, is often treated with painkillers like aspirin, ibuprofen, or paracetamol with Vitamin C supplements and plenty of bed rest. Allow me to go slightly go off track here and talk about vitamin C supplements for a little bit. Vitamin C is a complex molecule with multiple proponents to it, such as J, K and P factors and tyrosinase (organic copper) to name a few. The outer layer of this whole vitamin is called ascorbic acid. This is what is sold in vitamin C supplements, the outer coating which is almost entirely useless. Can ascorbic acid help with infections, possibly but the point I'm trying to make is to try to take Vitamin C from foods instead of supplements. Since fruits that are marketed as being high in Vitamin C, including but not limited to oranges, limes, and lemons, contain varying amounts of Vitamin C depending on the species, it can be tempting to overdo it and eat more oranges than necessary. As we covered previously, this actually leads to a significant increase in the amount of sugar eaten, which leads to the overproduction of insulin and can be harmful to the immune system, making it harder to recover from infections like the flu. Of course, when dealing with any kind of infection, it is important to get a wide range of vitamins including Vitamin A, D and B vitamins.

Let's consider a different type of recovery for a moment. Going to the gym or doing any form of exercise is a pastime for some and a wellbeing practice for others. Doing yoga helps with the mobility of the joints, cardio training helps the metabolism and resistance training burns calories while strengthening muscles and bones. After an intense workout, your body goes through a cooldown period where it processes the demands asked of it. This is part of the reason why some people enjoy a protein shake or "post workout electrolyte solution" after a workout. These can help accelerate your recovery time because, to use the electrolyte solution as an example, your body loses a lot of electrolytes through sweat. Electrolytes are simply compounds, such as salt and sugar. Delayed onset muscle soreness (also known as DOMS) happens in the hours after a tough workout or a long run. As the name implies, it's a deep-set soreness that can make itself known the day after a workout. This soreness can be treated with topical solutions, although the best form of treatment is done through prevention in the form of proper nutrition. Since plant-based diets do not have many naturally occurring sources of protein, recovery time takes longer and fatigue begins to set in much sooner than with a conventionally balanced diet.

One misconception about taking on a plant-based diet is that vegetarians and vegans do not experience food poisoning. This is not true. Food poisoning is another umbrella term simply referring to any illness that can be linked to food. Lacto-ovo vegetarians, for example, can get salmonella from eggs. Plant foods can also become contaminated through excessive use of chemical fertilizers and pests while still being grown. In the food industry, chemical substances such as antibacterial cleaners can contaminate food that is being prepared for service. If you were to go into a large, commercial kitchen, you would see a set of color-coded tongs. Typical coding is red for raw meat, green or tan for vegetables and fruits, blue for fix, yellow for cooked meat, and black or white for bread products. Malpractice in some commercial kitchens can lead to the wrong equipment being used on different foods. For example, red tongs being used on seafood and blue tongs being used on vegetables. Cross-contamination is a real possibility in the food industry, which is why government "red tape" is so stringent.

Hair

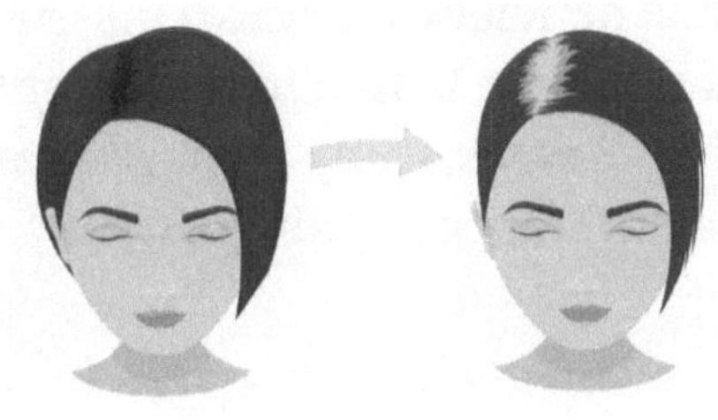

Among dermatological complaints, you might not expect conditions like alopecia and male pattern hair loss to receive mentions. A lot of things can cause people to lose their hair. Stress, for example, causes trichotillomania or excessive hair pulling. In women, polycystic ovary syndrome (PCOS) triggers the same gene that causes male pattern hair loss but in women, resulting in thinning hair and eventually baldness. Neither of these is caused by a plant-based diet, I'm just using them as well-known examples. Another cause of hair loss, as you may have guessed, is the lack of nutrition from a proper diet. It might surprise you to learn that your hair follicles actually have a very high metabolism. They are a major consumer of energy because of how much they use to keep growing. On average, hair grows at a rate of 2-3 inches per month with a healthy diet.

Recent studies examining the effects of mineral and vitamin supplements showed just how much the hair needs in order to grow. In one study, which explored different mineral and vitamin deficiencies, iron deficiency anemia was explored as a potential cause of hair loss. This theory actually dates back to 1963 and has since been evaluated, focusing on iron deficient women with a few recent studies looking at men. Many of these studies, both for men and women, have identified that iron does play a role in the health of hair. Therefore, we can assume that a lack of iron in the diet can result in unhealthy hair. Shedding is a natural part of the hair's lifecycle but, when it gets extremely brittle and unhealthy, it will start to fall out of its own accord. Another potential mineral deficiency is zinc. This theory is relatively new and has not been tested to the extent that iron deficiency has, but a 12 week study showed that zinc supplementation made a difference in hair growth.

Conclusion

A plant-based diet does have its benefits but these benefits are vastly outweighed by a series of negative side effects experience in the long run. Vitamin and mineral deficiencies are the root cause behind a variety of health complications, including heart disease. These deficiencies can also cause dental problems like tooth decay and plaque build up. Skin problems, including breakouts of acne and even dehydrated skin, can also arise as a result of a plant-based diet. Recovering from illnesses such as the flu or injuries, like broken bones, can take much longer, with treatments being heavily reliant on supplementation in order to speed up recovery time. Of course, everybody is different. While someone might experience some of these symptoms, someone else might see those symptoms knocking on their door much earlier.

In the next chapter, we are going to look at how to maximize nutrition from a plant-based diet. As promised in a previous chapter, we are going to explore how to minimize antinutrients as well as how best to manage macronutrients.

CHAPTER 7: HOW TO GET THE MOST OUT OF A PLANT-BASED DIET

Despite their inadequacies, plant foods can still be a part of your daily diet. If you enjoy the crunchy texture of carrot sticks with some hummus, some roasted broccoli with your salmon, or a nice hot apple pie for dessert, that is perfectly fine. By now, I hope you understand that carrots, broccoli, and apples, among other plant foods, are not the superfoods they are purported to be. However, some interesting things happen to plant foods when they are cooked or treated in certain ways. Take the apple in your apple pie. This type of apple is most likely a Granny Smith, a variety known for being tart and a little bitter. Apples are acidic, though not as acidic as a lemon or a grapefruit. This is because apples contain aromatic molecules. When cooked, these molecules break down and are converted into sugar. Apples, like Granny Smith, also tend to retain more flavor, although they lose more nutrients during the cooking process.

If you remember back in Chapter 4, we covered the antithesis of the nutrient: the antinutrient. For a quick recap, antinutrients act in such a way that your digestive system gets handicapped and becomes unable to absorb some nutrients from the food we eat. The absorption of iron, for example, can be inhibited by lectins. Lectins are a type of antinutrient found in beans, soybeans, and peanuts. Lectins are such a problem with regard to nutrition that a popular hypothesis is that it might be the root cause of the anaphylactic response to the top eight allergens: dairy, egg, wheat, soy, peanuts, tree nuts, fish, and shellfish. One study evaluated the lectin content of pulses, lentils, and beans, and identified that dietary lectins can induce an allergic reaction. Lectins do play a small role in body fat regulation, although it is more likely that they can cause obesity through leptin resistance. Leptin is a hormone made in the adipose tissue and acts as a regulator of energy.

Methods For Reducing Antinutrients

It is entirely possible to reduce the amounts of antinutrients in your plant foods. Antinutrients will always be present in your food. Much like sugar, they are everywhere and impossible to avoid. By making a few simple changes to your daily dietary habits, you can change the way your body absorbs nutrients. You may be familiar with the saying, "abs start in the kitchen." This saying refers to the fact that diet has more of an effect on one's health than exercise. On this same principle, I would like to amend it to "Good health starts in the kitchen." Part of this involves fostering a good relationship with your food. While a plant-based diet is not optimal, I recognize that not everyone would be able to embark on my diet and would still want to consume a variety of plants. Some people simply prefer to eat plants and I would like to offer some ways that can supercharge your food's nutritional value.

We're going to look at a variety of methods. They are all quite simple, though some require a little more work than others. For example, soaking beans overnight requires less work than growing your own plant foods from seed.

Soaking

You may have noticed that, in some health food stores and even grocery stores, you can buy packages of dehydrated beans. Dehydrating beans like kidney beans, chickpeas, and black turtle beans allows for a longer shelf life and this process has been used for thousands of years. Some estimates suggest that humans have been enjoying beans as a staple for up to 10,000 years, although some evidence suggests that this might be a conservative estimate. Approximately 7,000 years ago, beans were first domesticated in southern Mexico and Peru where climate patterns made it difficult to herd livestock for food purposes. For this reason, beans became a staple in both regions. 7,000 years later, and the British enjoy them on toast while Americans debate whether they belong in a batch of chilli.

For this method, I'm going to continue with the example of beans. Soaking beans in liquid either in the refrigerator or at room temperature for up to 8 hours can have a drastic effect on the texture, taste, and nutritional value of the bean. On the topic of nutritional value, most antinutrients are water soluble. This means that when they are introduced to water, they simply break apart and dissolve into the water. Antinutrients like lectins and phytic acid can be removed this way. It's even safe to boil the beans in the liquid they were soaked in because the antinutrients will not reform. However, it is recommended that you rinse the beans in order to remove excess starch and to preserve the texture of the beans themselves. The antinutrients that might remain are trace amounts and so negligible that you do not need to worry about them. Depending on the product, some suggest soaking for 12 hours is enough, while others say soaking can last for a few days and even a week or two. Usually, soaking for weeks on end also results in the fermentation of the food, creating a product with very minimal amount of antinutrients.

Canned beans have already been through the soaking and boiling processes, although be mindful of the liquid they come canned in. It could be full of salt and sugar, adding more calories and sodium to your diet. If you buy canned beans, make sure you read the nutritional info and rinse them before use. This will get rid of excess starch and any sodium or residue from being canned.

Boiling

Applying a steady amount of heat to plant foods in the form of boiling can degrade nutrients to the point that they are either inactive or have dissolved completely. As we saw in the above example, most antinutrients are water soluble. Boiling plant foods like carrots or potatoes can act as a sped up form of soaking since it applies heat, which speeds up dissolution. This is a particularly useful method to reduce protease inhibitors and lectins. One study looked at the effects of a combination of soaking and boiling on antinutrients in pigeon peas and cowpeas. The study showed that after an 80 minute stint of boiling, the two different types of pea showed a reduction of tannins by an average of 69%, while lectin was reduced by 79%.

Moving on from peas and beans to look at vegetables, one of the more common vegetables cited as a "great source of iron" is the leafy green. Leafy greens still contain antinutrients such as oxalates. A similar study showed that the reduction of oxalates in leafy greens can vary between 19-70% depending on how long they are boiled for and the temperature of the water they're being boiled in. Unfortunately, the boiling process does not seem to work on phytic acid. Phytic acid has heat resistant qualities, which makes it immune to this particular method of cooking. To reduce phytic acid, stick to soaking overnight or longer.

Fermentation

This method is particularly useful against phytates, enzyme inhibitors, and lectins. Fermentation is simply the process of allowing the chemical breakdown of substances in food to occur. This can be through bacteria, like with the fermentation of cheese, with yeast, as with the fermentation of breads, or the setting of milk to become yogurt. Fermentation has a lot of benefits. It allows bread to rise when baking and it adds a lot of probiotic properties to yogurt. This helps to improve your gut and intestinal flora, allowing for an easier digestion process.

Fermentation can significantly reduce phytic acid, enzyme inhibitors, and lectins because the bacteria or yeast consume the carbohydrates which form them, subsequently degrading the antinutrient. Most plant foods can be fermented, like apples can be fermented to make hard cider. However, grains like oats and wheat are most commonly fermented. Both are milled, which helps to break apart the compounds that form the antinutrients. When combined with fermentation, the bioavailability of nutrients is made much stronger.

Growing Your Own

This method of reducing antinutrients will, undoubtedly, take the longest depending on the type of crop you want to grow and the amount of space you have to grow it. Growing your own plant foods is a big commitment and requires a great deal of study and understanding when it comes to the individual plants you would like to grow. Tomatoes, for example, require a lot of phosphorus in order to grow efficiently and now every backyard has enough room to grow stalks of corn. Even Brussels sprouts can take up to two years to reach the stage where their buds can be shaved off and eaten. Trees can take up to 7 years, depending on the variety, to produce fruit and you have to take your climate into consideration. A warm, southern climate is ideal for growing avocados and lemons while a cooler climate is great for apples.

Growing your own fruits and vegetables also offers you a degree of freedom over what you are eating. Creating your own compost pile creates a hands-on source of nutrition for all the plants you intend to grow and can even cut down on food waste. Instead of throwing your food scraps into the garbage disposal, you can allow them to decompose naturally and even the local wildlife will "approve of" your compost. When it's ready, the compost will be full of earthworms, which will assist with decomposition and create a more nutrient-dense compost. You could even invest in a mechanical composter which separates the liquid from the solids. Neither liquid nor solid compost is inherently better than the other, although they do have their purposes. Mixing solid compost with soil and allowing it to mingle for a couple of weeks before planting allows the soil to become more nourished. Planting your seeds or pre-grown plants in these soil beds will only improve your plants' chances of survival.

Commercial farming focuses on producing higher yields, which can inhibit the quality of the plant foods being grown. Breeding plants to create higher yields often costs a lot in terms of nutritional quality as well as destroying the integrity of the soil, as we covered at the start of this book. By growing your own plant foods, you can cut back on your carbon footprint (if that's of concern to you), as well as grow enough for yourself and, potentially, share with family and friends. Growing your own food garden is also a fun and relaxing hobby, and you can really dig in deep by getting to know your own food.

Frozen Foods

Freezing is a method of food preservation that aims to extend the shelf life of certain foods. This method was first popularized by Sir Francis Bacon in 1626 when, as the story goes, he bought a chicken and packed it full of snow while on his way home. The modern method does not require packing whole chickens full of snow. The freezer in your kitchen maintains a steady temperature below 0 degrees Fahrenheit (-18 degrees Celsius). Professional kitchens aim to keep their freezers between 5-0 Fahrenheit (-15-18 Celsius) because this helps to preserve their frozen stocks.

Fruits and vegetables that you find in the freezer aisle are a good alternative to fresh fruits and vegetables. A 2015 study examined the effects of the freeze-thaw cycle on foods that are abundant in the Nigerian diet. The plant foods were primarily leafy green vegetables because not only are they a staple of the Nigerian diet, but they are a key source of some nutrients. What this study found was that freezing and thawing the food under investigation had no initial effect on nutritional quality. Fresh vegetables which were frozen within an hour of harvest retained the same level of nutrients after thawing as they had prior to being frozen.

One of the chemical processes that occurs as a result of freeing is the inactivation of specific enzymes. Your stomach contains certain enzymes that aid in the digestion of food. Plant foods also contain enzymes. Any living organism will have enzymes as part of its system because they help with the vital processes of life. If you leave a box of strawberries out on the kitchen counter at room temperature for a couple of days and then check on them, their condition will have deteriorated. This is because of oxidation and the enzymes within them. A bag of frozen strawberries, on the other hand, can last for up to 6 months to a year in the freezer before developing "freezer burn." When frozen, the enzymes are inactive. They are not in the right conditions to rot the food. Freezing can also kill a small amount of bacteria that could have otherwise degraded the food even more.

Some textural changes do occur as a result of freezing, although they are nothing to be concerned about. Freezing causes the water molecules to expand and crystallize. As the food thaws out the texture becomes softer because it loses moisture. This can also be due to the way it's thawed. If you thaw frozen vegetables completely before cooking and treat them as if they are fresh, their texture will not change. However, if you cook them straight from frozen at a higher temperature than you would for fresh vegetables, they will become soft and unpalatable. The key is to treat them as if they are fresh from the beginning and cook them low and slow with a little less water and just a pinch of salt with your favorite seasonings.

Buy Organic

Taking a trip to your local farmer's market will not only boost the local economy and save on your carbon footprint a smidge but will give you access to healthier plant foods. Buying organic is primarily better for the soil. As we explored earlier, modern farming practices quickly become detrimental to the plants, the soil, and the overall environment. Local growers implement polycultural farming techniques and grow on a much smaller scale than industrial farms. One of the reasons for this is that they use fewer chemical pesticides. A misconception about organic farming is that there are no pesticides used when crops are grown. This is not the case. Wherever there are crops, there are pests and where there are pests, there are methods to get rid of those pests. Industrial farms will use large batches of synthetic pesticides while organic farmers will use pesticides that are natural in origin. I want to make something clear: everything is a chemical. If something says "free from chemicals," it's likely a marketing tactic. This is part of the draw to the organic market. The chemicals used in organic pesticides, such as neem oil or eucalyptus spray, are natural in origin. They are not created in a lab with the sole purpose of wiping out pests. Instead, they kill the pests while also replenishing the soil.

The soil is healthier as a result of organic farming. This is due to less stress on the structural integrity of the soil in addition to the implementation regenerative agriculture or holistic management practices. Organic farming is also more sustainable and encourages the local population to get involved through allotment gardening. This leads to a variety of changes in energy consumption and overall environmental welfare. For example, when we looked at the downsides of industrial farming at the start of this book, we saw that local water supplies become polluted as a direct result of chemical pesticides and fertilizers. Organic farming reduces this and makes use of biodegradable sources, which are more water soluble and are easier to separate when the water is filtered for consumption.

Apple Cider Vinegar

You may have seen apple cider vinegar touted as an "all-natural miracle weight loss supplement." Apple cider vinegar can help you digest your food but it does nothing to help you lose weight fast. The reason I bring it up is because it can actually help you digest your food by acidifying your stomach and break down the antinutrients in plant foods before they have the chance to bind themselves to nutrients and steal them from you. Another way apple cider vinegar can be helpful is its effects on acid reflux and GERD. Studies into its efficacy are still ongoing but, from the information we have, we know that it is safe to consume when diluted with water. There is little scientific evidence that apple cider vinegar can assist with bloating but the theory is that its assistance with digestion can alleviate symptoms in the long term.

Conclusion

There are quite a few ways you can reduce the antinutrient content of certain plant foods. Soaking for 12 hours minimum is recommended but it can also be left to soak for several days. Boiling is basically soaking but fast forwarding while also breaking it down with heat. Though it might sound disgusting, fermenting or basically rotting some plant foods is an option to reduce antinutrients. Taking on the hobby of growing your own food is a good personal challenge as well as being rewarding once your plants come into harvest.

Get comfortable as we dive into our last chapter. We will be discussing my recommendations for a proper diet as well as other good alternatives.

CHAPTER 8: SO WHAT SHOULD WE BE EATING?

Diet is not the only ingredient for good health. Exercise is also important and so is mental wellbeing. For the moment, we are going to stick with diet, although physical health will also factor into the discussion. When considering the diet that is best for you, you need to take into consideration any intolerances or allergies you might have. Someone who is allergic to shellfish might not want to take on a pescatarian diet, for example. Somebody like me, who struggled for a month eating a plant-based diet, would most likely benefit from an omnivorous or majority carnivorous diet. Personally, I vouch for the ketogenic diet because it has worked best for me, although I do know people who struggled with it just the same as I did with being vegetarian. No two people are the same and neither are any two diets. There is no "miracle" diet and there is no such thing as "good" food or "bad" food. Anyone who comes along promising you that his special diet or product will make you lose 20lbs or more in 10 days is most likely attempting to sell you a scam. The key to maintaining good health is to strive for balance and wellness.

Nobody is the same. Someone may experience nasty symptoms after eating a certain food while others just simply don't. It's hard to create a fix all diet that can help everyone. Diet is a personal thing that must be custom made by you. For me, I feel better on a meat based keto diet with plenty of fats with a bit of carbs. If you feel tired or still hungry after a meal, try raising the calorie content of your meals. The objective is to feel satisfied after a meal while trying to get a variety of micronutrients in the process. Everyday, you should track how you feel after certain meals to try and find what you can tolerate and what you cannot. Notice if you feel depressed or irritable after eating something. Usually, if these symptoms occur, you are most likely intolerant to these foods.

Personally, I follow a high-carb ketogenic diet heavily focused on meat products. I'm a pretty lean and fit guy and eating a higher amount of carbs makes me feel a bit better. In terms of carbs, I usually eat pasta, bread (I recommend sourdough) and potatoes. Though I have found myself eating a variety of vegetables because of friends and family, but I usually stick around cucumbers, zucchinis, broccoli, potatoes, lemons and celery just to name a few. I chose these vegetables not because they are healthier or less inflammatory than other plant foods, but mostly just because of the fact that I can tolerate them and enjoy them. I understand that not everybody is the same, therefore I will also provide a little bit of information on other diets.

Types Of Diets

There are many diets out there. You will probably think of the "trendy" or "fad" diets that become popular as a result of good marketing. However, I want to give a brief overview of a few different diets in the more literal sense. That is to say, I just want to talk about the different kinds of food humans eat in order to sustain themselves. All a diet is is a method of nourishing your body.

Ketosis

The principal aim of the keto diet is to force the body into a state of ketosis. That is to say, it forces your body to start burning fat for energy as opposed to sugar and carbohydrates. For this reason, the diet is a high-fat, moderate-protein and minimal-carbohydrate diet. Fermented foods such as yogurt, sour cream, cheese, sauerkraut, and kimchi are commonly eaten as part of this diet. Even though sauerkraut and kimchi are plant-based foods, the fermenting process allows them to break down the antinutrients present and develop not only more flavor but more nutritional value. Lean poultry, most commonly chicken and turkey, is also allowed as well as red meat.

Ketosis can be quite restrictive, depending on your approach to it. Most people cut out every single carbohydrate they can think of: pasta, bread, pizza, cake, fruits, and vegetables. If it's a carb, they get rid of it. However, the keto diet actually has a lot of room for development and variety.

There's a reason keto cookbooks exist, after all, and that reason is that there are four types of keto diet:

- **Standard Keto**
- **Cyclical Keto**
- **Targeted Keto**
- **High Protein Keto**

Standard keto is pretty self-explanatory. Typical macros for this diet are 70% fat, 20% protein, and 10% carbohydrates. If you're brand new to keto, this is the type of structure I would recommend following since it gives your body a chance to adjust to a new way of eating and a new way to process and burn energy. **Cyclical keto** is similar to an 80:20 plan. For example, you might have five "ketosis" days where you follow the standard keto macros but implement two "high carbohydrate" days to allow your body a little cheat day. **Targeted keto** is much more flexible. In this form of the diet, you can increase or decrease your carbohydrate intake depending on your workouts. For example, if you have a heavy cardio day at the gym, you can have an extra slice of toast or bowl of pasta salad to give your body an extra burst of energy; if you have a heavy weight training day, you might cut back on the carbs and focus more on a high-protein version of ketosis. Lastly, **high protein keto** follows a similar structure to the **standard keto** plan but with an emphasis on protein. Standard macros for this version of the diet would look something like this: 60% fat, 35% protein, and 5% carbohydrates. This version is followed by "veterans" of the keto diet, so people whose bodies are used to burning more fat than usual.

This diet has a variety of health benefits. In addition to the lowered risk of heart disease and its benefits relating to diabetes, ketosis is currently being investigated as a potential treatment for cancer. Although this is something of a wildcard, the theory is that providing the body with an alternative energy source—for example, fat instead of carbohydrates—in combination with standard chemotherapy and other treatments, it could help improve recovery rates and allow treatments to work more effectively. At the time of writing, this research is relatively new and should be taken with a pinch of salt until further evidence has come to the surface. Even so, this is an interesting development and should be watched closely.

I will go into a little more detail about how to begin this diet later. My experience following the keto diet has given me some insight in how to make this dietary conversion more successful to those who are new.

GAPS (Gut and Psychology Syndrome)

The Gut and Psychology Syndrome (GAPS) diet is an elimination diet designed for people who experience digestive distress. It was created by Dr Natasha Campbell-McBride, a British neurologist. Her philosophy for this diet is that the food we eat has more profound effects on the brain than we might think. The diet removes all of the foods which the body has difficulty processing, and slowly reintroduces them over the course of two years.

This is not a diet to take lightly because it can take up to two years to effectively implement and complete. For reference, there are six introductory stages to complete before you can move onto the full diet regimen.

1. Anyone experiencing severe digestive symptoms (diarrhea, abdominal pain, bloating, etc.) should eat homemade soup stocks made fresh from meat, poultry and fish. Probiotics, including kefir, and herbal teas are also allowed at this stage.
2. Add organic raw egg yolks, homemade ghee, fermented fish. This builds up on the proteins and amino acids present in the previous stage. A little salt and some fresh herbs are allowed.
3. At this stage, you can add nut butters, whole eggs, cooked and fermented vegetables and ripe avocados back into your diet alongside high-quality probiotic supplements.
4. Roasted and grilled meats and cold-pressed olive oil, with fresh pressed vegetable juices and nut flours, are added back in to supplement the carbohydrates present in the previous stage.
5. Fresh pressed fruit juice is now allowed to supplement the vegetable juice from the previous stage, in addition to raw vegetables and even apples.
6. Finally, all raw fruits from the GAPS-approved list are allowed back into the diet. Berries, bananas and coconut are allowed although dried fruits and nuts and seeds should be eaten in moderation.

Once these six introductory stages have been completed, you can move on to the full GAPS diet regimen. This diet was created to help people with gut induced psychological issues. As covered in the previous chapter, the gut health and the brain health have a huge connection. This diet focuses on healing the digestive tract to then heal the mind.

Flexitarian

"Flexitarian" is a portmanteau of "flexible" and "vegetarian." This diet is also referred to as "semi-vegetarianism." A flexitarian diet is predominantly plant-based but with the flexibility to allow for meat. Depending on the person practicing a flexitarian diet, there is room for up to 28 oz of lean meat (including poultry, fish, and red meat) per day. People who do not enjoy the taste or texture of meat but do not want to cut it out entirely might be interested in following this diet. Similarly, this diet would be an option for anyone who wants to include more plant foods in their diet but does not want to give up animal products.

The flexitarian diet, as well as "plant-based" dieting' proclaims to have a few benefits. To give an example, the meat processing industry accounts for large amounts of carbon dioxide gas which has a significant effect on the environment. One of the most common reasons to take on a vegetarian diet is to reduce your carbon footprint. When practicing a flexitarian diet, you can cut down your carbon footprint. The theory behind this is that it saves on natural resources and cuts down on carbon emission. Though all of this sounds good and all, it's not entirely true. I will be discussing this common false argument in future books. You definitely don't want to miss out on those!

However, there are a few downsides to this diet. Just the same as with the vegetarian diet, the risk of developing iron deficiency anemia, B12 deficiency is still a possibility. Although iron deficiency anemia is less likely due to the presence of heme iron through lean meat, this is still something to be aware of. Speak to a medical professional about any concerns or find some supplements which work for you. Just like with the keto diet, the key to this diet is planning your meals and keeping track of what you are eating.

Carnivore

The carnivore diet is an entirely animal-based diet featuring nothing but red meat, poultry, fish, seafood, eggs, dairy products and honey excluding all foods that come from plants. Some of the proposed health benefits of this diet include blood sugar regulation, improved mood and weight loss. There is limited research into these purported health benefits although plenty of testimonial evidence exists in support of it. There are currently no studies in regards of the effects of a long-term carnivore diet but we can take a look at our past. We now know that some primitive tribes had a diet that was heavily focused on animal products, such as the Maasai of Africa and the Alaskan/Canadian Inuits. Since they lived in an environment with very poor access to plant foods, they mostly ate meat and lived long and healthy lives. In fact, the Maasai are known for their excellent physical, height and strength.

Since this diet removes practically all inflammatory foods, it gives a chance for your body to recover. In fact, it gives the chance to your body to recover from almost all diseases. Some claim to have healed from their autoimmune diseases and type 2 diabetes. One popular story is the one from Jordan Peterson himself as well as his daughter. He claims to have healed from depression, cirrhosis, sleep problems and more as well as being intellectually sharper. The interview can be viewed on the Joe Rogan's podcast on YouTube. Tons of success stories have also made their appearance recently on the internet.

You might be interested trying this diet in the short-term if you are on a cut, need to up your intake of protein or heal from a certain disease. Since this diet lacks dietary fiber, some proponents of the diet recommend adding probiotic, unfruited yogurts and prebiotic to keep feeding your gut microbes.

The Ketogenic Diet: Some Tips

Ketosis and the ketogenic diet have a pretty unique origin. As early as 500 B.C.E., utilizing ketosis for short periods of time has been used in the treatment of epilepsy. From the 1920s onwards, it became a medical treatment alongside medications, such as sodium valproate. With the increase in antiepileptic medications, the ketogenic diet fell out of use and eventually became a common treatment in pediatric hospitals. Part of the reason it was such an effective treatment was because it mimicked fasting and it was noted that seizures were less severe during treatment. As it fell out of medical popularity, it was destined to go mainstream. A combination of celebrity endorsement, scientific backing and social media fueled the keto revolution. It soon became a popular diet for bodybuilders and fitness enthusiasts worldwide.

I would like to take this opportunity, in the last chapter, to offer some advice. Ketosis has worked wonders for me and others all around the world. It has gotten something of a bad reputation because "keto warriors" have created the impression that you have to be obsessed with your food in order to get the most from it. This is not always the case. Unless you are on an elimination diet like GAPS, any diet is flexible. Keeping track of your macros and calories can be a challenge. Ketosis, especially if you are doing it with a specific goal in mind like weight loss or muscle building, has a specific set of guidelines. Even with these guidelines, the variety of food offered surprised me when I first started.

If you are struggling to start, keep these things in mind: high fat, moderate protein and low carb. Those are common practice, but it can get hard to keep track. Inspiration in the form of cookbooks and recipe websites are always within reach. As with any diet, you should consult a dietitian before attempting to start keto.

The keto diet comes with a lot of health benefits. Since it mimics fasting, your metabolism taps into fat instead of glucose for fuel, which supports weight loss. Another way in which keto supports weight loss is by reducing hunger hormones, such as ghrelin. Ghrelin is the hormone which signals hunger and is often triggered by low blood sugar. Keto meals, as you will discover, are made of much more substantial fare than plant-based meals. We have already established in a previous chapter that the body takes longer to break down protein. For this reason, blood glucose tends to stabilize. As a result, hunger hormones, such as ghrelin, take longer to release and stimulate the hunger response. Let's put this into context. A 2013 meta-analysis studied 13 separate controlled trials that compared different diets. Among these was the ketogenic diet. On average, the participants who were on the keto diet lost around 2lbs more than any other diet. A more recent study of a larger sample size, and following a slightly longer period, showed an average weight loss of 5lbs.

Conclusion

Plants are not what they seem to be. While a common household plant adds some color and character to your home, the plants you eat as part of your daily diet offer little to no nutritional value. Many factors go into this. First and foremost, the incessant breeding of plants to favor increased yield over increased nutritional content contributes to a variety of health problems rooted in malnutrition. A lack of Vitamin D, for example, means that the bones and teeth are unable to absorb calcium for remineralization. As a result, osteoporosis and tooth decay are common complaints among people who follow a strict plant-based diet. While the body can synthesize Vitamin D from the sun, a diet lacking in cholesterol can still lead to a Vitamin D deficiency since cholesterol is a precursor. Most vitamins and minerals are only found in large amounts in animal foods. Amino acids can be found in plant-based sources but the body will have a hard time breaking them down and synthesizing them into the proteins it requires. Since the body can only make 11 out of the 20 amino acids it requires, it relies on a proper diet to gain them. Without these amino acids, many vital processes cannot take place.

A healthy diet is all about sourcing the right foods. This does not mean striving to get the exact right amount of iron every single day nor does it mean trying to eat a meal that has been weighed down to the ounce. All this means is that you feel comfortable with the food you are giving your body and that you trust that your body knows what to do with it. Because a lot of plant-based protein sources are so full of carbohydrates, fat, and salt, the body struggles to process them.

While it is alarming that plant foods are not the vital sources of nutrition they are claimed to be, the necessity of monocultural farming needs to be addressed. Polycultural farming has its downsides, which are rooted in the years of practice and knowledge required for it to be effective. Regenerative agriculture is the answer to the problems caused by conventional farming practices. Perhaps the most immediate change we would see would be in the structure of the soil. Soil takes some structural damage with every planting season. Although this cannot be avoided, it can easily be repaired by allowing the soil to rest and be nourished. Since regenerative agriculture or holistic management has the space to allow for crop rotation, the soil will gain different nutrients with each planting. Livestock is kept on farms regardless of the farming practice, so allowing the livestock to graze would allow the soil to become rich from the nutrients provided by natural manure. This would cut down on the dependency of synthetic chemical fertilizers. Pests will still be a problem but they will not be nearly as prevalent as they are on monoculture farms.

I hope that this book has given you a good understanding of why plants are not what they seem to be. This is something I have been passionate about for a long time and, from my own experience, I can say that the problems we face in terms of nutrition are rooted in the way we view our food.

Please, take a few days to process the information I have presented to you and start taking steps to a healthier, more nutritious, lifestyle.

A community

If you want to be part of a likeminded community, you can join our facebook group Nutrition Delusion where we share plenty of interresting facts and edifying stories. My books will also be available at a discounted price if you join the facebook group.

Plus, you can directly go to my website:
www.nutritiondelusion.com
to get your very own free copy of my <u>7 lies About Food</u> list. All you have to do is enter your name and email address and you will receive your free copy in your emails. Don't forget to check in your junk mails :)

Also, please don't forget to **leave a review** on Amazon. Every review helps authors like me reach more people.

References

8 Signs and symptoms of vitamin A deficiency. (2018, June 2). Healthline. https://www.healthline.com/nutrition/vitamin-a-deficiency-symptoms#TOC_TITLE_HDR_3

9 Signs you may have vitamin K2 deficiency. (2014, October 6). Dr. John Day. https://drjohnday.com/9-signs-you-may-have-vitamin-k2-deficiency/

10 Antinutrients to get out of your diet immediately. (n.d.). Dr. Axe. https://draxe.com/nutrition/antinutrients/

Apple cider vinegar for bloating: Does it work? (2019, October 31). www.medicalnewstoday.com. https://www.medicalnewstoday.com/articles/326866

Arnarson, A. (n.d.). *How to reduce antinutrients in foods*. Healthline. https://www.healthline.com/nutrition/how-to-reduce-antinutrients

At-a-glance / brochure - 2011 Meat eaters guide. Meat eater's guide to climate change + health. Environmental Working Group. (n.d.). www.ewg.org. https://www.ewg.org/meateatersguide/at-a-glance-brochure/

AZoCleantech. (2013, January 31). *What are the environmental benefits of crop rotation?* AZoCleantech.com. https://www.azocleantech.com/article.aspx?ArticleID=369

Barre, A., Damme, E. J. M. V., Simplicien, M., Benoist, H., & Rougé, P. (2020). *Are dietary lectins relevant allergens in plant food allergy?* Foods, *9*(12). https://doi.org/10.3390/foods9121724

Berg, J. M., Tymoczko, J. L., & Lubert Stryer. (2002). *Proteins are degraded to amino acids*. Nih.gov; W H Freeman. https://www.ncbi.nlm.nih.gov/books/NBK22600/

Berg, J. M., Tymoczko, J. L., & Lubert Stryer. (2016). *Important derivatives of cholesterol include bile, salts, and steroid hormones*. Nih.gov; W. H. Freeman. https://www.ncbi.nlm.nih.gov/books/NBK22339/

Berg, J. M., Tymoczko, J. L., & Stryer, L. (2002). *The biosynthesis of amino acids*. Biochemistry. 5th Edition. https://www.ncbi.nlm.nih.gov/books/NBK21178/

Berrazaga, I., Micard, V., Gueugneau, M., & Walrand, S. (2019). *The role of the anabolic properties of plant- versus animal-based protein sources in supporting muscle mass maintenance: a critical review*. Nutrients, *11*(8), 1825. https://doi.org/10.3390/nu11081825

Bioavailability of plant-based proteins. (n.d.). www.foodunfolded.com. https://www.foodunfolded.com/article/bioavailability-of-plant-based-proteins

Bourre, J. M. (2005). *Where to find omega-3 fatty acids and how feeding animals with diet enriched in omega-3 fatty acids to increase nutritional value of derived products for human: what is actually useful?* The Journal of Nutrition, Health & Aging, *9*(4), 232–242. https://pubmed.ncbi.nlm.nih.gov/15980924/

Breen, L., & Churchward-Venne, T. A. (2012). *Leucine: a nutrient "trigger" for muscle anabolism, but what more?*. The Journal of Physiology, *590*(9), 2065–2066. https://doi.org/10.1113/jphysiol.2012.230631

Brown, M. J., Ameer, M. A., & Beier, K. (2021). *Vitamin b6 deficiency*. PubMed; StatPearls Publishing. https://

pubmed.ncbi.nlm.nih.gov/29261855/

Chai, W., & Liebman, M. (2005). *Effect of different cooking methods on vegetable oxalate content.* Journal of Agricultural and Food Chemistry, *53*(8), 3027–3030. https://doi.org/10.1021/jf048128d

Delany, A. (n.d.). *Is soaking dried beans overnight really necessary?* Bon Appétit. https://www.bonappetit.com/story/soaking-dried-beans-overnight-necessary

digestion-of-gluten. (2019, October 8). Dr. Schär Institute. https://www.drschaer.com/us/institute/a/digestion-gluten

Dirt poor: have fruits and vegetables become less nutritious? (2011). Scientific American. https://www.scientificamerican.com/article/soil-depletion-and-nutrition-loss/

Environmental consequences of modern production agriculture : How can alternative agriculture address these issues and concerns. (n.d.). www.eap.mcgill.ca. https://www.eap.mcgill.ca/MagRack/AJAA/AJAA_1.htm

Fine Cooking Editors. (2015, September 3). *The science of apples.* FineCooking; Fine Cooking. https://www.finecooking.com/article/the-science-of-apples

Food. (2019, September 12). *These "natural" foods were actually man-made.* Healthygem. https://www.healthygem.com/food/these-natural-foods-were-actually-man-made/?view-all&chrome=1

Freed, D. L. J. (1999). *Do dietary lectins cause disease?* BMJ : British Medical Journal, 318(7190), 1023–1024. https://www.ncbi.nlm.nih.gov/pmc/articles/PMC1115436/

Frequent tillage and its impact on soil quality / Integrated crop management. (2019). Iastate.edu. https://crops.extension.iastate.edu/encyclopedia/frequent-tillage-and-its-impact-soil-quality

Gerster, H. (1998). *Can adults adequately convert alpha-linolenic acid (18:3n-3) to eicosapentaenoic acid (20:5n-3) and docosahexaenoic acid (22:6n-3)?* International Journal for Vitamin and Nutrition Research. Internationale Zeitschrift Fur Vitamin- Und Ernahrungsforschung. Journal International de Vitaminologie et de Nutrition, 68(3), 159–173. https://pubmed.ncbi.nlm.nih.gov/9637947/

Gupta, R. K., Gangoliya, S. S., & Singh, N. K. (2013). *Reduction of phytic acid and enhancement of bioavailable micronutrients in food grains.* Journal of Food Science and Technology, 52(2), 676–684. https://doi.org/10.1007/s13197-013-0978-y

https://www.facebook.com/thepaleomom. (2019, May 8). *Genes to know about: Vitamin a conversion genes ~ The paleo mom.* The Paleo Mom; The Paleo Mom. https://www.thepaleomom.com/genes-to-know-about-vitamin-a-conversion-genes/

Hunt, J. R. (2003). *Bioavailability of iron, zinc, and other trace minerals from vegetarian diets.* The American Journal of Clinical Nutrition, 78(3), 633S639S. https://doi.org/10.1093/ajcn/78.3.633s

Insider, S. G., Business. (n.d.). *These 6 common vegetables are actually all the same plant species.* ScienceAlert. https://www.sciencealert.com/these-6-common-vegetables-are-actually-all-the-same-plant-species

Is flour bad for you? Modern grain vs. ancient grain. (2020, May 15). Full of Days. https://everydayfull.com/is-flour-bad-for-you/

Kasarda, D. D. (2013). *Can an increase in celiac disease be attributed to an increase in the gluten content of wheat as a consequence of wheat breeding?* Journal of Agricultural and Food Chemistry, *61*(6), 1155–1159. https://doi.org/10.1021/jf305122s

Kerri-Ann Jennings, MS, RD. (2017, March 10). *What is a pescatarian and what do they eat?* Healthline; Healthline Media. https://www.healthline.com/nutrition/pescatarian-diet

Klement, R. J. (2019). The emerging role of ketogenic diets in cancer treatment. *Current Opinion in Clinical Nutrition and Metabolic Care, 22*(2), 129–134. https://doi.org/10.1097/mco.0000000000000540

Lewis, T. (2018). *Here's what fruits And vegetables looked like before we domesticated them.* ScienceAlert. https://www.sciencealert.com/fruits-vegetables-before-domestication-photos-genetically-modified-food-natural

Link, A. (n.d.). *Lectins.* Allergy Link. https://www.allergylink.co.uk/allergy-blog/2018/07/03/lectins/

Mawer, R. (2018). *The ketogenic diet: A detailed beginner's guide to keto.* Healthline. https://www.healthline.com/nutrition/ketogenic-diet-101

Molina-López, J., Florea, D., Quintero-Osso, B., de la Cruz, A. P., Rodríguez-Elvira, M., & Del Pozo, E. P. (2016). *Pyridoxal-5'-phosphate deficiency is associated* with *hyperhomocysteinemia regardless of antioxidant, thiamine, riboflavin, cobalamine, and folate status in critically ill patients.* Clinical Nutrition (Edinburgh, Scotland), 35(3), 706–712. https://doi.org/10.1016/j.clnu.2015.04.022

Mousa, M. (2020, May 12). *Fruits, nuts, and vegetables you did not know were man-made.* Cooking with Lubna. https://www.cooksfood.net/post/fruits-nuts-and-vegetables-you-did-not-know-were-man-made

Mullens, A., & Scher, B. (2019, April 28). *Sinking our teeth into the carnivore diet: what's known, what's not.* Diet Doctor; Diet Doctor. https://www.dietdoctor.com/low-carb/carnivore

National Geographic Society. (2012, October 9). *Dead zone.* National Geographic Society. https://www.national-geographic.org/encyclopedia/dead-zone/

National Institutes of Health. (2017). *Office of dietary supplements - vitamin D.* Nih.gov. https://ods.od.nih.gov/factsheets/VitaminD-HealthProfessional/

NHS Choices. (2019). *Leaky gut syndrome.* NHS. https://www.nhs.uk/conditions/leaky-gut-syndrome/

Onwuka, G. I. (2006). *Soaking, boiling and antinutritional factors in pigeon peas (cajanus cajan) and cowpeas (vigna unguiculata).* Journal of Food Processing and Preservation, 30(5), 616–630. https://doi.org/10.1111/j.1745-4549.2006.00092.x

Pesticide contamination of farm water sources. (n.d.). www.omafra.gov.on.ca. http://www.omafra.gov-.on.ca/english/engineer/facts/15-001.htm#:~:text=Surface%20runoff%20water%20picks%20up

Raji, A. O., Akinoso, R., & Raji, M. O. (2015). *Effect of freeze-thaw cycles on the nutritional quality of some selected Nigerian soups.* Food Science & Nutrition, 4(2), 163–180. https://doi.org/10.1002/fsn3.271

Rebekah. (2019, April 4). *Alternatives to Tilling Your Spring Garden.* J&R Pierce Family Farm. https://jrpierce-familyfarm.com/2019/04/04/alternatives-to-tilling-your-spring-garden/

Reynolds, R. D. (1988). *Bioavailability of vitamin B-6 from plant foods.* The American Journal of Clinical Nutrition, 48(3), 863–867. https://doi.org/10.1093/ajcn/48.3.863

Rosell, M., Appleby, P., Spencer, E., & Key, T. (2006). *Weight gain over 5 years in 21,966 meat-eating, fish-eating, vegetarian, and vegan men and women in EPIC-Oxford.* International Journal of Obesity, *30*(9), 1389–1396. https://doi.org/10.1038/sj.ijo.0803305

Ruiz-Tagle, S. A., Figueira, M. M., Vial, V., Espinoza-Benavides, L., & Maria, M. (2018). *Micronutrients in hair loss.* Our Dermatology Online, *9*(3), 320–328. https://doi.org/10.7241/ourd.20183.25

Seidel, K. (2020, June 10). *History of dried beans – How it all started.* Cablevey® Conveyors. https://cablevey.com/history-of-dried-beans-how-it-all-started/

Selective breeding and gene technology - Eduqas - Revision 1 - GCSE Biology (single science) - BBC bitesize. (2019). BBC Bitesize. https://www.bbc.co.uk/bitesize/guides/zqftrwx/revision/1

Shapiro, J. (2007). *Hair loss in women.* New England Journal of Medicine, 357(16), 1620–1630. https://

doi.org/10.1056/nejmcp072110

Shapiro, J., Wiseman, M., & Lui, H. (2000). *Practical management of hair loss.* Canadian Family Physician, 46(7), 1469–1477. https://www.cfp.ca/content/46/7/1469.short

Sharp, A. (2020, June 24). *Are antinutrients safe? Lectins, oxalates, phytates and more.* Abbey's Kitchen. https://www.abbeyskitchen.com/are-antinutrients-safe-lectins/

Smith, M. (2020, January 9). *Are Vegans Depressed?* Medium. https://psychologymarc.medium.com/are-vegans-depressed-7eda14c5d4e5

Streit, L. (2019, December 13). *The flexitarian diet.* Healthline. https://www.healthline.com/nutrition/flexitarian-diet-guide#downsides

Streit, L. (2019, August 26). *All You Need to Know About the Carnivore (All-Meat) Diet.* Healthline; Healthline Media. https://www.healthline.com/nutrition/carnivore-diet

Tan-Shalaby, J. (2017). *Ketogenic diets and cancer: Emerging evidence.* Federal Practitioner : For the Health Care Professionals of the VA, DoD, and PHS, 34(Suppl 1), 37S42S. https://www.ncbi.nlm.nih.gov/pmc/articles/PMC6375425/

Tello, M. (2018, February 22). *Diet and depression - Harvard Health Blog.* Harvard Health Blog. https://www.health.harvard.edu/blog/diet-and-depression-2018022213309

The benefits of garden-to-table produce versus supermarket varieties. (n.d.). GardenTech.com. https://www.

gardentech.com/blog/gardening-and-healthy-living/garden-to-table-goodness-and-nutrition

The traditional four-step method. (n.d.). Bean Institute. https://beaninstitute.com/the-traditional-four-step-method/

Tonstad, S., Butler, T., Yan, R., & Fraser, G. E. (2009). *Type of vegetarian diet, body weight, and prevalence of type 2 diabetes.* Diabetes Care, *32*(5), 791–796. https://doi.org/10.2337/dc08-1886

US EPA. (2019, January 28). *The sources and solutions: Agriculture | US EPA.* US EPA. https://www.epa.gov/nutrientpollution/sources-and-solutions-agriculture

Vin Kutty. (2010, March 23). *Omega-3 deficiency symptoms.* OmegaVia. https://omegavia.com/deficiency-symptoms/

Vitamin k2 — A little-known nutrient can make a big difference in heart and bone health. (n.d.). www.todaysdietitian.com. https://www.todaysdietitian.com/newarchives/060113p54.shtml

Watanabe, F., & Bito, T. (2017). Vitamin B12 sources and microbial interaction. *Experimental Biology and Medicine, 243*(2), 148–158. https://doi.org/10.1177/1535370217746612

West, H. (2017, July 23). *The GAPS diet: An evidence-based review.* Healthline; Healthline Media. https://www.healthline.com/nutrition/gaps-diet

What every vegan should know about vitamin b12. (2019). The Vegan Society. https://www.vegansociety.com/resources/nutrition-and-health/nutrients/vitamin-b12/what-every-vegan-should-know-about-vitamin-b12

What is a pescatarian diet? (2019). BBC Good Food. https://www.bbcgoodfood.com/howto/guide/what-pescatarian-diet

What Is the Carnivore Diet? Benefits, Risks, Food List, More | Everyday Health. (n.d.). EverydayHealth.com. https://www.everydayhealth.com/diet-nutrition/diet/carnivore-diet-benefits-risks-food-list-more/

What Is The Carnivore Diet: 5 Reasons Why This Diet Is Nonsense. (2020, October 15). Atlas Biomed Blog | Take Control of Your Health with No-Nonsense News on Lifestyle, Gut Microbes and Genetics. https://atlas-biomed.com/blog/carnivore-diet-myths/

What's wrong with modern wheat. (2019). GRAINSTORM. https://grainstorm.com/pages/modern-wheat

Wheless, J. W. (2008). History of the ketogenic diet. *Epilepsia, 49 Suppl 8*, 3–5. https://doi.org/10.1111/j.1528-1167.2008.01821.x

Which form of vitamin a is most absorbable? Beta-carotene or retinol? (2016, April 20). https://www.onlineholistichealth.com/betacarotene-retinol/

Wild/natural fruit vs. modern/cultivated fruit. (n.d.). www.beyondveg.com. https://www.beyondveg.com/billings-t/fruit-table/wild-cultiv-fruit-1a.shtml

Yi, Y., Li, X., Jia, J., Guy Didier, D. N., Qiu, J., Fu, J., Mao, X., Miao, Y., & Hu, Z. (2020). *Effect of behavioral factors on severity of female pattern hair loss: An ordinal logistic regression analysis.* International Journal of Medical Sciences, 17(11), 1584–1588. https://doi.org/10.7150/ijms.45979

New Study-Vitamin K2 Lowers Coronary Heart Disease Risk (May 28, 2020). https://www.nattopharma.com/new-study-vitamin-k2-lowers-coronary-heart-disease-risk/

Gut microbiome and depression: what we know and what we need to know. https://pubmed.ncbi.nlm.nih.gov/29397391/

Effects of fecal microbiota transplant on symptoms of psychiatric disorders: a systematic review

https://pubmed.ncbi.nlm.nih.gov/32539741/